ROBOTICS RESEARCH AND TECHNOLOGY

DUTY-SPLIT APPROACH IN ROBOTIC SURGERY

ROBOTICS RESEARCH AND TECHNOLOGY

Robot-Age Knowledge Changeover
Rinaldo C. Michelini
2009. ISBN: 978-1-60692-905-6
2009. ISBN: 978-1-60876-390-0 (E-book)

Duty-Split Approach in Robotic Surgery
Rinaldo C. Michelini, Silvia Frumento and Roberto P. Razzoli
2010. ISBN: 978-1-61668-232-3
2010. ISBN: 978-1-61668-457-0 (E-book)

ROBOTICS RESEARCH AND TECHNOLOGY

DUTY-SPLIT APPROACH IN ROBOTIC SURGERY

RINALDO C. MICHELINI,
SILVIA FRUMENTO
AND
ROBERTO P. RAZZOLI

Nova Science Publishers, Inc.
New York

Copyright © 2010 by Nova Science Publishers, Inc.

All rights reserved. No part of this book may be reproduced, stored in a retrieval system or transmitted in any form or by any means: electronic, electrostatic, magnetic, tape, mechanical photocopying, recording or otherwise without the written permission of the Publisher.

For permission to use material from this book please contact us:
Telephone 631-231-7269; Fax 631-231-8175
Web Site: http://www.novapublishers.com

NOTICE TO THE READER

The Publisher has taken reasonable care in the preparation of this book, but makes no expressed or implied warranty of any kind and assumes no responsibility for any errors or omissions. No liability is assumed for incidental or consequential damages in connection with or arising out of information contained in this book. The Publisher shall not be liable for any special, consequential, or exemplary damages resulting, in whole or in part, from the readers' use of, or reliance upon, this material.

Independent verification should be sought for any data, advice or recommendations contained in this book. In addition, no responsibility is assumed by the publisher for any injury and/or damage to persons or property arising from any methods, products, instructions, ideas or otherwise contained in this publication.

This publication is designed to provide accurate and authoritative information with regard to the subject matter covered herein. It is sold with the clear understanding that the Publisher is not engaged in rendering legal or any other professional services. If legal or any other expert assistance is required, the services of a competent person should be sought. FROM A DECLARATION OF PARTICIPANTS JOINTLY ADOPTED BY A COMMITTEE OF THE AMERICAN BAR ASSOCIATION AND A COMMITTEE OF PUBLISHERS.

LIBRARY OF CONGRESS CATALOGING-IN-PUBLICATION DATA

Michelini, Rinaldo C.
> Duty-split approach in robotic surgery / Rinaldo C. Michelini, Roberto
>Razzoli.
>   p. ; cm.
> Includes bibliographical references and index.
> ISBN 978-1-61668-232-3 (softcover)
> 1. Surgical robots. I. Razzoli, Roberto. II. Title.
> [DNLM: 1. Surgery, Computer-Assisted. 2. Robotics. WO 505 M623d 2010]
> RD73.S785M53 2010
> 617'.9178--dc22
>   2010002979

Published by Nova Science Publishers, Inc. ✢ New York

CONTENTS

Preface		vii
Abstract		ix
Chapter 1	Introduction	1
Chapter 2	Computer-Assisted Surgery	5
Chapter 3	The Split-Duty Approach	17
Chapter 4	Augmented Reality Actions	25
Chapter 5	Conclusion	43
References		49
Index		53

PREFACE

Mini-invasive surgery deserves increasing attention to lower post-operative stays in hospitals and to lessen fall-off complications. This new book is devoted to surgical robotics, with a focus on technology and design issues of the remote-mode operation assistants. The investigation leads to define the technical characteristics of a CRHA, co-robotic handling appliance, to be purposely developed, to support the duty-split approach surgical planner.

ABSTRACT

Mini-invasive surgery deserves increasing attention to lower the post-operative stay in hospital and to lessen the falls-off complications. This leads to the new trends in robotics, to provide help for safe and accurate remote manipulation, as innovative opportunity of integrated computer-aided implements. Out of front-end haptic effectors, the background support is turning to inclusive on-duty functions, e.g., surgical planners, operation assistants, etc., making possible the rethinking of protocols, based on the anthropocentric dimensions, to progressively embed the innovations offered by the micro- and nano-technologies.

The state of the arts, already, shows impressive new attainments, notably, towards expanding the operation versatility of successful achievements (e.g., the forth arm in daVinci® system) and looking at ambient intelligence tricks, to widen the on-duty flexibility, so that scope-driven alternatives, out of man-handling reach, are conceived and performed.

The chapter brings in the surgical robotics, with focus on technology and design issues of the remote-mode operation assistants. The investigation leads to define the technical characteristics of a CRHA, co-robotic handling appliance, to be purposely developed, to support the duty-split approach surgical planner. The expected peculiarities and advantages are outlined, including the analysis of the operation potential of special-purpose contrivances (e.g., the automatic changing device of the surgical tools) and of scope-driven enhancers (e.g., the exploration of the intervention theatre, *IT*). The presentation, thereafter, addresses example developments, with explanatory intention, taking, as starting points, also, projects performed with the co-operation of other robot laboratories in Munich and in Paris. The CRHA concept is investigated in connection with the DLR KineMedic® arm (developed by the Munich laboratory), and with the LRP prototypal mini-arm (built by the Paris laboratory). The main features of the example CRHA design are summarised for the two developments, with constructive details, especially, turned on the actually available DLR KineMedic® arm. The overall comments consider the mini-invasive robotic surgery as factual intervention practice in the near future, and the duty-split approach, supported by the CRHA technology, as valuable aid for the human-robot co-operation, according to the "best-of-skills" concept, fully supporting the intervention responsibility, under the direct surgeon's control.

Keywords: robot surgery, minimal-invasive surgery, co-robotic equipment.

ACRONYMS

STAC, surgical tool automatic change.
CRHA, co-robotic handling appliance.
IT, intervention theatre.
MIRS, minimally invasive robot surgery.
OR, operating room.
OT, operating table.

Chapter 1

INTRODUCTION

The robotics is multidisciplinary technology, developed to perform tasks in co-operation with, or without direct human intervention. Anthropomorphism is a reduced issue when:

- the tasks to be performed are coherently defined, so that their programming and control are fully described by protocols and reliably implemented in the intervention theatre;
- the expected duties are out of standard human capabilities because of performance complexity and accuracy requirements, hostile surroundings and safety risks , etc. and require sound and rescaled solutions.

The robotics follows, with the typical features of: functionally driven presets; task programming and up-dating; oversight of surroundings and intelligence; as well as autonomous management within the given specifications. Surgical robots, similarly, follow this evolution, moving from mainly anthropomorphic configurations, to progressively more duty-driven geometry.

The switch from man-like to duty-driven devices is deemed to occur in parallel with the development of minimally invasive robot surgery, **MIRS**, [Lum, 2006; Konietschke, 2004; Seibold, 2005]. Radical advances are expected to have an impact on micro-surgery in deep, narrow sites in the body; these provide the most difficult challenges for minimally invasive surgery; examples are: neurosurgery with poor visibility due to blood or cerebrospinal fluid; microsurgery in the outer wall for oesophageal, an area not accessible with the traditional endoscope through the mouth; and the like. Similarly changes are expected with the micro- and nano-technologies, when end-effectors, scaled for very localised interventions, are offered, with accuracy and handling capabilities beyond standard human range.

The robotic achievements are technology-driven with results connected to:

- information infrastructure: data acquisition, handling, vaulting, transmission, validation, processing, etc. are continuously expanding options supported by the ICT, and effective new computer tools ceaselessly appear to support remote supervision and control. Tele-medicine is a fully acknowledged technology [Reintsema, 2004; Guthart, 2000; Intuitive Surgical, 2005], while remote-surgery has chiefly experienced noteworthy accomplishments [Rosen, 2006];
- execution effectors: specialised tools and fixtures are possibly the most challenging research opportunity today, closely tied to human scale [Cepolina and Michelini, 2004]. In the future, surgeons will continue to deal with standard size devices; inner-body equipment will evolve in timely fashion toward micro- and nano-apparatuses, as soon as effective new solutions are conceived and made available [Farokhzad, 2006; Silva, 2007].

This twofold fall-out, basically, leads to the complementary developments of «computer integration» and of «functionally-driven instrumentation», together leading to «computer-aided surgery».

The biggest research challenge is the simultaneous need for micro-manipulation in local interventions, and gross motions at the handling level. This conflict is resolved by the master/slave option, to perform micro-manipulation by miniature slaves, scaled from natural size motion by the master controller. This format, however, needs especially implemented information infrastructures, with due focus on the direct and indirect potential of the effectors, but, also, enhanced attention to the opportunities for computer integrated support.

These supporting opportunities are the enablers to expand robotics in planning and implanting surgical interventions more accurately and less invasively, each time confining the effectors to narrow spaces. We expect to see the emergence of four complementary roles:

- surgical planning will integrate accurate patient specific models, surgical process optimization, and a variety of execution protocols

permitting the plans to be fulfilled accurately, safely and with minimal invasiveness;
- surgical effectors will evolve progressively new operating tools, conceived as special-purpose task-driven devices (out of the anthropomorphic scale) and based on the emerging micro- and nano-technologies;
- surgical ambient-intelligence will support the man/robot interface to assure the transfer of the surgeon's expertise, know-how and proficiency, towards the local, minimally invasive, intervention theatres;
- surgical assistants will work co-operatively with human surgeons in carrying out precise, highly effective and reliable surgical procedures, always assuring continuous monitoring and supervision.

Over time, these roles will merge into a broad family of aids that integrate multi-disciplinary information, into actions of interventional medicine. On this basis «computer integration» for surgery is a fast growing field with proven accomplishments.

Chapter 2

COMPUTER-ASSISTED SURGERY

2.1. METHODS AND TECHNOLOGIES

The discussion on the computer-assisted surgery, further to methods and technology prospects, needs to be addressed as already well established opportunity. Indeed, robot surgery is established practice, possessing noteworthy equipment, quite effective and reliable.

With minimally invasive robot surgery MIRS in mind, the role of the ancillary aids (actuators, sensors, etc.) is exactingly linked with the interface technologies (ambient intelligence, etc.), being instrumental, the two together, for enabling highly innovative and more conservative intervention protocols. We face, here, one of the situations, where the deep understanding of the really needed duties and of the actually available means, brings in suggestions, coherent for pace-wise improvements. Let, first, shortly review the current methods, before summarising possible technological developments.

The deep sites micro-surgery applies with resort to the catheter procedure. The trocar is positioned with insertion of the guide wire and is threaded through the organs, to the site to be operated. The guide wire is withdrawn, and the slave micro-manipulator is inserted along the tube to the chosen site. The endoscope and one or more slave manipulators, as needed by the intervention, may be inserted in the same way. Then, the remote handling is used to accomplish the micro-surgery by the slave manipulation in the restricted space, while monitoring provides the images from the endoscope. In principle, the operation progression depends on the master/slave effectiveness; therefore, the interface technology deserves great attention, as through it the devices are controlled and managed to expand front-end versatility and generate operation flexibility.

One significant problem with endoscope surgery, whether robotically assisted or free-hand, is the effect of entry port location on the surgical site handling dexterity. Several authors [Jacobs et al. 2003; Taylor et al., 1999] have addressed this subject, but there is much more research to be done, both, in planning and in developing robots with higher distal dexterity.

Another significant problem is motion of the anatomy being operated upon, especially in cardiac cases, and several groups are exploring approaches to accommodate such motion [Detter et al., 1999; Damiano et al. 2000]. The manipulation limits imposed by human hand tremor and restricted ability to feel and control very small forces, together with the constraints of on-duty microscopes, have led a number of researchers to investigate the microsurgery robotic augmentation. Several systems have been developed for remote handling, using passive input device for the operator control. Guerrouad and Vidal [Guerrouad and Vidal, 1989] describe a system designed for ocular vitrectomy, in which the mechanical manipulator is build to follow curved tracks to maintain fixed centre of rotation. An alike micro-manipulator is used for acquiring physiological measurements in the eye by an electrode. Similarly, an ophthalmic surgery manipulator, built by Jensen *et al.* [Kumar et al., 2000], aims at retinal vascular microsurgery, and is capable of positioning instruments at the surface of the retina with submicron precision. While useful test device, this system does not reach enough motion range to be useful for general-purpose microsurgery. Also, the lack of force sensing prevents the study of force/haptic interfaces in fulfilling the microsurgical tasks.

Actually, the enhanced interfacing functions need careful validations. Today protocols, almost exclusively, manoeuvre by sequential schedules, so that, even when multiple-task engagement is planned, stop and delay are included to maintain the focus on the pace-wise intervention fulfilment. This corresponds to the unique responsibility of the in-charge surgeon, who avoids the resort to assistants, unless as auxiliary side-matches or as exceptional alarm interference. The master/slave option is, thus, featuring technology, especially when intuitive motion ties are exploited, to create the friendly correspondence between the in situ actuation and the remote controller.

Many microsurgical robots [Miroir, et al., 2008; Wei et al. 2006; Fine et al., 2009] are based on the force-reflecting master slave concept. This allows the operator to grasp the master manipulator and apply forces. The forces, measured on the master, are scaled and reproduced at the slave; if unobstructed, they cause the slave to move accordingly. Likewise, the forces, encountered by the slave, are scaled and reflected back to the master. This configuration allows position commands from the master to result in a reduced motion of the slave, and for forces encountered by the slave to be enlarged at the master. The force-reflecting master-slave microsurgical system provides the surgeon with increased accuracy and enhanced perception, but drawbacks exist to such a design. Complexity and cost are primary snag, linked with the need to duplicate the manipulation devices, one for the master and one for the slave.

The master-slave setting and the co-operative force-controlled trimming nicely emphasise the extension of the surgeon's own dexterity, with, however strong anthropocentric bent. Several groups are beginning to explore indirect, more sophisticated ways to use the robot's capabilities to assist the surgeon. Much of this work extends the "active constraint" idea used by Davies *et al.* in the knee surgery system, to develop sensor-mediated "virtual fixtures" that constrain the robot's motion or create haptic feedback directing the surgeon to move the effectors in a desired direction. More complex behaviours have, as well, been modelled and implemented for prototype interactive tasks, aiming at optimised case solutions.

The choice shows that, even if many micro-effectors are there at the intervention theatre, the co-operation falls within the governing capabilities of the in-charge surgeon (out of the recalled side-matches and distress actions). The fact distinguishes computer-integrated surgery, from traditional computer-integrated industrial applications, where process automation develops free from direct anthropocentric conditioning knots. Here, the research needs to tackle with more subtle opportunities, that range at two layers:

- forefront features, e.g., artificial fingers haptic abilities, straight steered by a remote man hand, co-operating with other instruments, steered by the second remote man hand;
- backdrop aids, e.g., on-process adapting the end-effectors location by co-robotic carriers, with simultaneous up- or down-scaling the monitored images, by ambient intelligence interfaces.

The duty-split approach affects the latter layer, but major up-grading is expected by synergy with the former. This approach is specifically dealt with in the chapter.

Once shortly figured out the duty-frame, the procedural outline gives further insight on technologies. The anthropocentric conditioning is, both, active and passive. At the master front-end, the surgeon shall operate in natural way, enhancing his sensorial capabilities within natural habits. At the slave side, the surroundings deals with a human body, having push, pull, shear and stretch limitations, directly reported to natural figures. Therefore, to ease the operation, the continuous interlacing of forefront features (the intervention headway) and backdrop aids (the check-and-adapt raise) permits to realize synergic effects to expand the reach of the surgeon's skill, reserving the all responsibility under his/her mastery.

The technologies to support these accomplishments, accordingly, have to deal with augmented degrees-of-freedom, at, both, forefront and backdrop. In the first case, we have, further to the effectors miniaturisation, the developments of articulated mini-probes, capable to shape and reshape during the intervention, to locate the front-tip with proper posture, nevertheless not damaging delicate organs along the penetration path-way. The snake-like mini-probes [Cepolina, 2005] can have passive self-shaping properties and, then, cannot bear tips applying active thrust. They can have active shaping abilities, mainly, with wire-driven external actuation. The mini-probes, with inner actuated joints, at the moment, face severe limitations, and only prototypal devices exist.

The augmented degrees-of-freedom at the backdrop are more easily implemented, as they represent quite conventional robotic architectures, not constraint by the contact with the living surroundings. The idea leads to robotic aids with co-operation, and is specially discussed in the present study. The functional redundancy requires a parallel steering logic, so that the end-effectors are able to accomplish the duty sequence, fixed by the intervention protocols, through alternative agendas, or by mixing different protocols. The steering logic might develop at several levels of complexity. With the today end-effectors and the (practically) sequential schedules, the augmented degrees-of-freedom, already, provide effective advantages at the level of surgical assistants, especially in connection with advanced ambient-intelligence. The study of the duty-split approach is, anyway, very important to start recognising the peculiarities of robotic aids with co-operation.

2.2. STATE OF ARTS EXAMPLES

The da Vinci Equipment

Perhaps, the most impressive achievements, today, belong to the Intuitive Surgery, with the widely used systems da Vinci®. The da Vinci® has a monolithic structure, with the recent advance given by the four-arm robot model, figure 1, and remote ergonomic console. Launched in April 2009, the da Vinci Si HD introduces Advanced 3D HD visualization with up to 10x magnification and an immersive view of the operative field, *EndoWrist®* instrumentation with dexterity and range of motion far greater than even the human hand, *Intuitive®* motion technology, which replicates the experience of open surgery by preserving natural eye-hand-instrument alignment and intuitive instrument control, *Dual-console capability* to support training and collaboration during minimally invasive surgery. The system allows the surgeon to use the fourth arm for key steps and manoeuvres during the operation, thereby decreasing the reliance on advanced assistant laparoscopic skills.

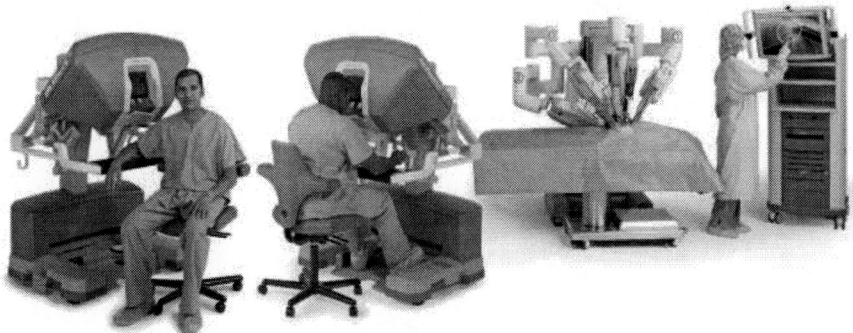

Figure 1. The four arms daVinci robot with governing dual console.

The Sensei® X Equipment

Hansen Medical proposes the Sensei X Robotic Catheter System a robotic catheter placement device, which uses a system of pulleys to navigate a steerable sheath for catheter guidance, figure 2. The Sensei X provides the physician with more stability and more force in catheter placement compared to manual techniques, allowing for more precise manipulation with less radiation exposure to the doctor, commensurate with higher procedural complications to the patient, including cardiac perforations, tamponade and femoral artery incurie. The Sensei X Robotic Catheter System, by translating human hands motions at the workstation to the control catheter inside the patient's heart, empowers accurate catheter placement.

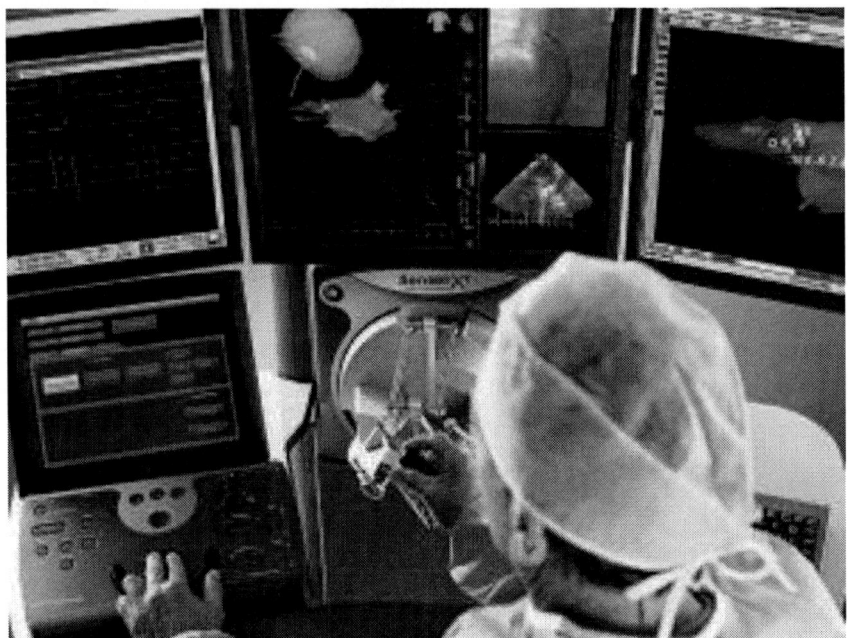

Figure 2. Sensei® X Robotic Catheter System.

The RoboDoc Equipment

The RoboDoc (previously marketed by Integrated Surgical Systems) now by CUREXO Technology Corporation, surgical system consists of the Orthodoc, a pre-operative planner, and the RoboDoc, a surgical tool, figure 3. The RoboDoc was developed in the 1980s and is currently used in hospitals in Europe. It is first used in total hip replacements and its use is now extended to revision hip replacement and total knee replacement. RoboDoc has been cleared by the U.S. Food and Drug Administration (FDA) for Total Hip Arthroplasty procedures, making it the only active robotic system cleared by the FDA for orthopaedic surgery.

The RoboDoc surgical system uses Computer Tomography to obtain structural information of the surgical object pre-operatively. The OrthoDoc allows the surgeon to construct a pre-operative bone-milling procedure. Before the bone-milling procedure, registration is conducted to match the pre-operative data with the physical location of the surgical object. In total hip replacement, RoboDoc is used to cut the femoral cavity precisely.

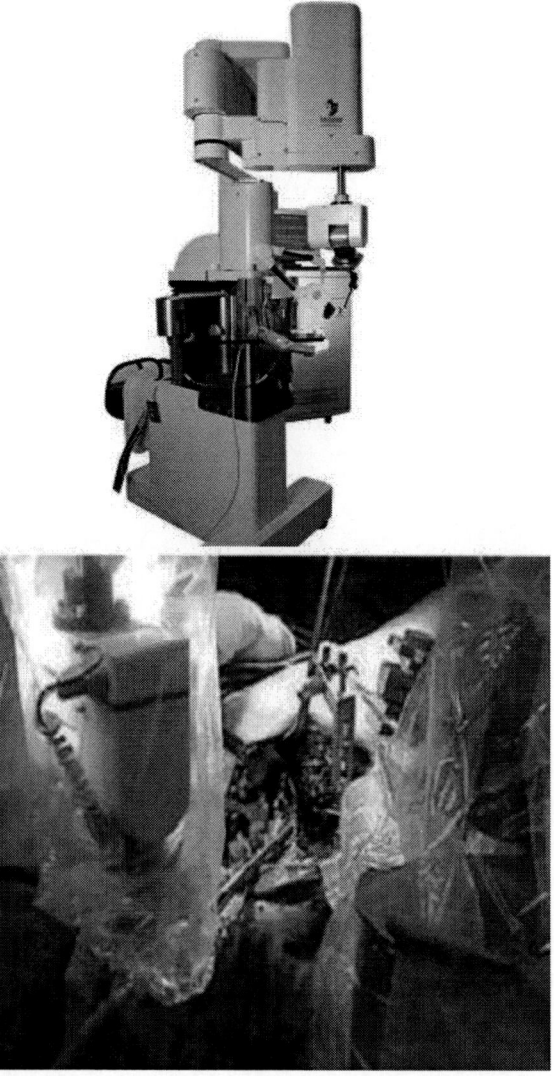

Figure 3. ROBODOC® system for hip and surgery by CUREXO Technology Corporation.

The Caspar Equipment

CASPAR robot is produced by U.R.S. Ortho GmbH & Co. KG, and is used for total hip, total knee and anterior cruciate reconstruction, figure 4. For complex reasons, the company has gone into liquidation in the last few years; however a lot of CASPAR robots are still active.

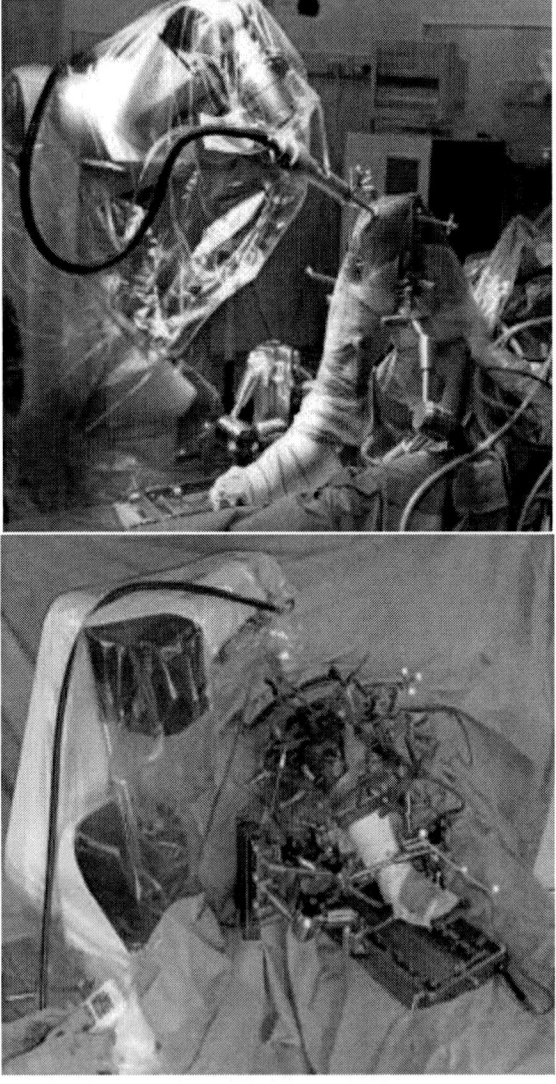

Figure 4. Caspar® system for hip and knee replacement.

The CyberKnife Equipment

The CyberKnife®, by Accuray, is a stereostatic radio-surgery system [Antypas C and Pantelis, 2008]: the 6 DoF serial robot is equipped with 6 linear accelerometers, figure 5; the stereoscopic image system automatically detects and locates the areas to be treated. The set-up avoids the resort to rigid frames, enhancing the patient comfort.

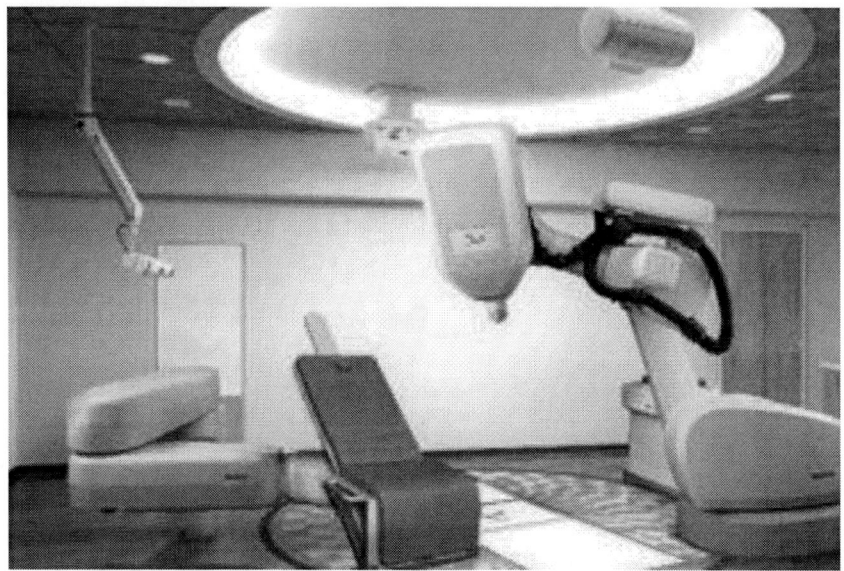

Figure 5. The CyberKnife® System.

The Naviot Equipment

A special purpose system is developed recently in Japan [Hashizume and Tsugawa, 2004] for laparoscope manipulation, Naviot™ (Hitachi, Tokyo, Japan), figure 6. This system is recognized as the first surgical robot ever developed in Japan. It is based on a five-bar linkage mechanism which has two independent motors on the bottom. In addition, the zoom-up mechanism of the laparoscope is applied to this manipulation system. The moving range was about 25° in both the vertical and horizontal directions. As of March 2004, it already performed laparoscopic surgery on 100 patients.

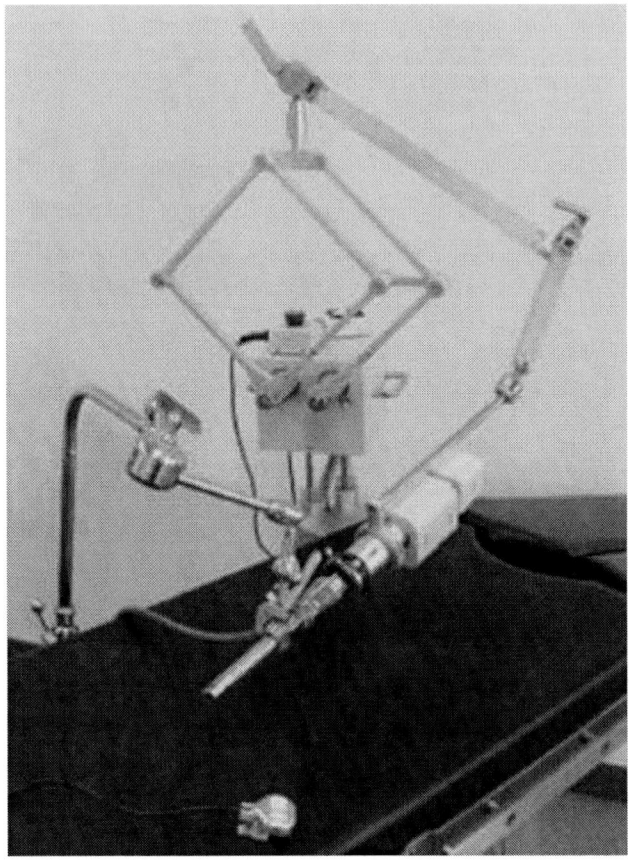

Figure 6. Laparoscope manipulator, Naviot™.

The Neuromate Equipment

Neuromate, figure 7, is distributed by Renishaw Mayfield, a subsidiary of Renishaw: it is the only robot CE marked for neuro-endoscopy and provides access to the ventricular system and in deep brain structures. Image-guided planning with a user-defined safety corridor and accurate manoeuvring with a remote control allow a single surgeon to perform accurate surgeries with a safer access and a firm instrument support. The system was cleared by FDA in July 1999 for use with a frameless head assembly, which is intended to replace the bulky conical frames worn by patients during brain surgery. The frameless system is a light plastic device that holds an ultrasound sensor, which relays signals to the surgical robot about the position of the patient's brain in relation to the robot arm.

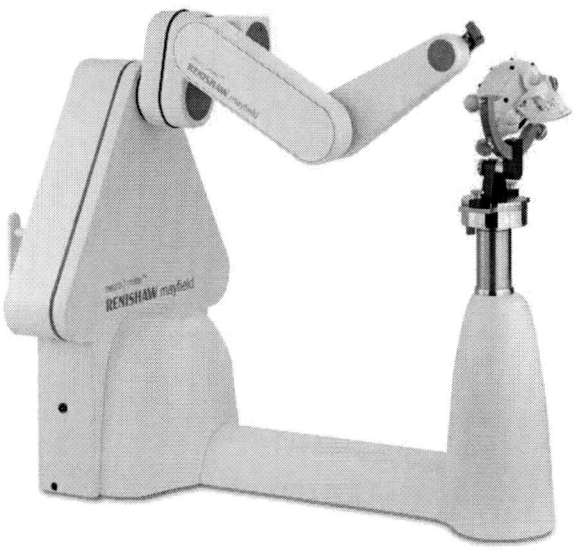

Figure 7. Neuromate system for brain surgery.

Chapter 3

THE SPLIT-DUTY APPROACH

3.1. METHODOLOGICAL PROSPECTS

The operation flexibility on the intervention theatre becomes urgent requisite, to expand the effectiveness and the reliability of the surgical robotics solutions. The demand can be tackled from different prospects. A systemic approach needs to move from the knowledge (previously recalled) prerequisites, to not disregard the foreground knowledge, when developing the instrumental proposal. Besides, the background knowledge assumes two distinct areas, depository of the medical, either, of engineering sciences. Then, the computer-assisted surgery expands as technology-driven option, to encompass:

- passive aids (navigation and aiming devices, enhanced restitution displays, etc.);
- supporting aids (action guided interventions, based on known strategies, finally enabled by the surgeon);
- autonomous aids (task sequences performed by the robot, under the watchful eye of the surgeon).

The information infrastructure, mainly, supplies passive aids and co-operates to the feasibility of autonomous or assisted actions. The execution effectors aim at replacing the human actors front-end actions, with benefits as for accuracy, daintiness, dexterity, efficiency, safety, size, versatility, etc., once the tools are optimised in terms of the duties to be fulfilled (and anthropocentric limitations are overrun).

Robotic surgery, according to the four complementary deployments (surgical planners, effectors, ambient-intelligence and assistants), offers the winning support for minimal invasiveness, by two means:

- the inherent handling effectiveness of the instrumental front-ends, joined to the remote control abilities;
- the functional extensions of the integrated interventions planned and ruled through ambient intelligence.

The anthropocentric approach mixes the two means, enhancing the tested surgeon's expertise, with higher handling accuracy, versatility, reliability and sensitivity. The deployment complementarity requires that, on one side, the conventional rules in designing *instrumental* robots, with account of the duty-driven functions, ought to be followed; and, the other side, the understanding of the intervention peculiarities has to develop as task-reliant surgeon's incumbency.

In the analysis, typical aspects in the minimal-invasive robotic-surgery are tackled in view of finding out by which ways computer-integration will affect the future trends, with emphasis on expected *instrumental* handling forecast. The remarks especially address the *hardware* components; similar prospects apply for the software aids, however, less conditioned by task-reliant limits and more exposed to operation schedules (e.g., function planning) and computer-driven innovations (e.g., ambient-intelligence). The *instrumental* handling aspects need to further distinguish the basic properties of the architectural lay-out (we propose the *split-duty* approach, to separately address arms positioning and effectors duties), from the evolution of the reference technologies (to keep the pace of innovation by carefully looking after the desired *functions* optimisation, by, e.g., modular built-ups [Bidaud et al. 2004]). The hints are merely a spur for further discussion, but proper acknowledgement of typical robot features seems a factual way to provide suggestions to innovate, also, in the medical fields, in keeping with the instrumental robotics philosophy.

Along these ideas, reliability and safeness are fundamental robot-surgery demands, as interventions apply on human beings, robotic rigs are in contact with patients (and staff), the responsible operators (surgeons, etc.) are not robot-experts, etc.; the instrumental aids, thereafter, need to grant complete transparency to the supplied function, with no bias of mechanical couplings, information handling, reconfiguration procedures, etc., that, possibly, occur. To that aim, a surgical device has always to comply with *overall* requirements:

no uncontrolled motions; bounded output forces/displacements; self-recovery end-effectors; constant surgeon's overseeing, and so on, making it clear that the built-in trustworthiness is unavoidable request.

These requests lead to *redundancy* in mobility, sensors and control, and to *recovery* in operation, actuation and intelligence. Different robotic architectures and functional strategies might be devised, such as the *split-duty* approach. This characterises by distinguishing:

- the auxiliary rigged frame, granting the correct positioning and feeding of the overall set-up, as specific rig of the surgery assistance;
- the front-end effectors, performing, after the in-body access of tools and cameras, the intervention under the direct surgeon's control.

The two together lead to the Co-Robotic Handling Appliance, **CRHA**, hereafter discussed providing details on the reference architectures and on the utilisation protocols. Each sub-system is hierarchically governed by the remote locations, following effective protocols, while the interfaced operators receive the sub-set of information at the selected *degree* of *immersion*, with suggestions of consistent (*vs.* not advisable) actions (under priority restrictions).

The robot augmentation features, then, are combined effect of the mechanical architectures and functional strategies, once the background knowledge (surgery expertise and ancillary engineering aids) is exploited. In fact, the *split-duty* approach, simply, provides a means for extra-redundancy in manipulation, and for higher reliability in task-progression, without implying the definition of specific surgical interventions, or the choice of given technological tools.

3.2. CO-ROBOTIC HANDLING APPLIANCE

The survey, now, addresses the *Co-Robotic Handling Appliance*, starting from the reference example architectures. The split-duty planning helps the computer-aided surgery, by allowing separate task-programming of the carrying rig, and of the front arms [Cepolina and Michelini, 2003; Frumento, 2006]. In the operation room, several layouts can be considered:

- floor base, carried by trolleys; as the characteristics of a monolithic structure result obviously different compared to individual trolleys, with individual vertical strokes to adjust the height of the arms;
- table base, expected to separately address each arm, granting the option to slide along the table edges and to provide individual vertical adjust as well;
- wall base, with transversal frame fixed on walls, carrying the arms in the centre of the room; a telescopic guide lifts and lowers the arms and a linear horizontal guide adjusts the location;
- ceiling base, above the patient, with the possibility to slide on the ceiling plane and to lower itself in order to reach the neighbourhood of the selected organ;
- patient base, with the robotic arms directly on the patient's body, when size and weigh allow it.

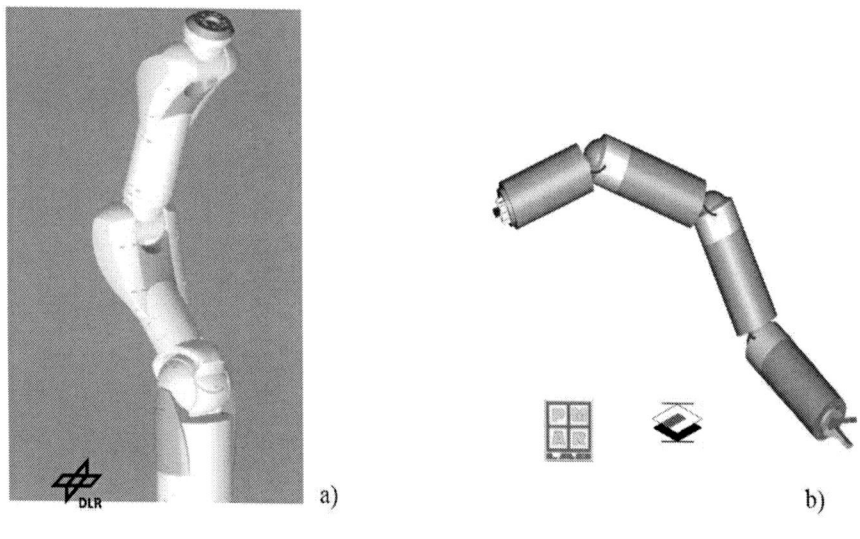

Figure 8. The DLR KineMedic® arm and the prototypal LRP mini-probe.

The **CRHA** is just an element in the split-duty approach, and, to better explain the prospected opportunities, two example developments are out-lined, taking, as robotic front-effectors, quite different equipment, such as the KineMedic® arm, figure 8a, developed at the DLR of Munich and now available with the KUKA industrial co-operation, and the LRP prototypal mini-probe, built and tested at the Paris laboratory, figure 8b. The first equipment is assumed to operate with table mount, paralleling three or four

KineMedic® arms. The second is at a very early experimentation stage, and is thought to work with patient mount. In both cases, the split-duty approach comes out as innovation towards computer-assisted surgery, in the lines of the present ideas.

The **CRHA** for the DLR arms is expected to have larger size and wider workspace, and can be conceived to, mainly, operate along sequential planning. In the LRP mini-probes case, the limited effectors workspace presumes more sophisticated control strategies, and the setting is affected by the request of proper task-mode co-operating options. The ceiling mount is chosen after proper investigation, summarised by the above recalled criteria. The choice allows the quick withdrawal of the robots from the *IT*, moving up to the room ceiling, typically free from equipment. Indeed, during the MIRS interventions, the need of switching to the traditional surgery could occur. Statistics show that approximately one out of one hundred times complications appear. In this case, the robot has to be quickly removed from the patient, and placed where it does not represent a barrier. The surgeon must leave the remote stand and perform the intervention in situ. It is, therefore, important that, at emergencies, the robot has a set-up that allows fast removal.

3.3. MINI-PROBE EFFECTORS

In the LRP mini-probe situation, the reference **CRHA** is noticeably lighter, figure 9. The prospected setting aims at four (or more) mini-probes, having the individual tips located on the same horizontal plane, nearby the positions of the trocars inserted in the patient's body. Up now, prototypal devices have been assembled, figure 9 b, and tested also in operative conditions [Sallé et al., 2004; Cepolina and Michelini, 2005].

The individual mini-probe is protected inside a case, from where it can spiral out, figure 9 a. Each case can independently rotate, to approach the best location, near the patient. The drums operate as 'dispenser', also providing guiding support during the mini-probe pulling out. The insertion, through the trocar, inside the body, is remotely governed.

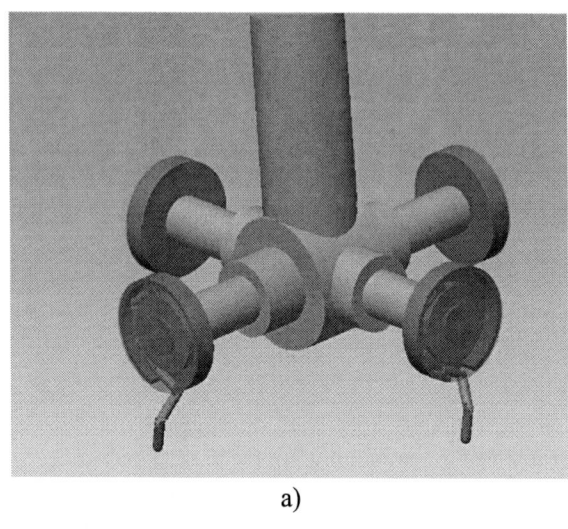

a)

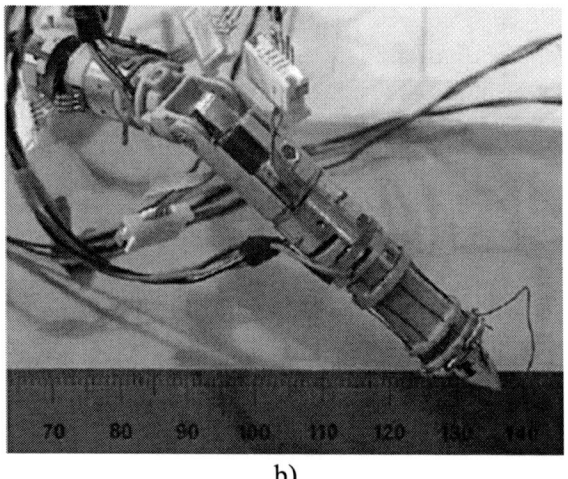

b)

Figure 9. The CRHA carrying four LRP mini-probes (a); test bench of the prototypal device (b).

3.4. CO-OPERATION SETTING

In the **CRHA** development, focus is kept on modularity, notably, to select the ceiling guides. The standard lay-out, figure 10, considers a telescopic pole, with the DLR arms appended to co-axially mounted revolving carriers, and with the superposed surgical-tool automatic change, **STAC**, equipment. The front and side views provide the details for the three DLR arms arrangement [Frumento et al., 2006].

The **CRHA** is deemed to become common complement in **MIRS**. Likewise, the *split-duty* approach reaches full deployment when the co-operation comes in as standard routine, re-thinking the on-duty protocols by the combined mobility of carrier and effectors.

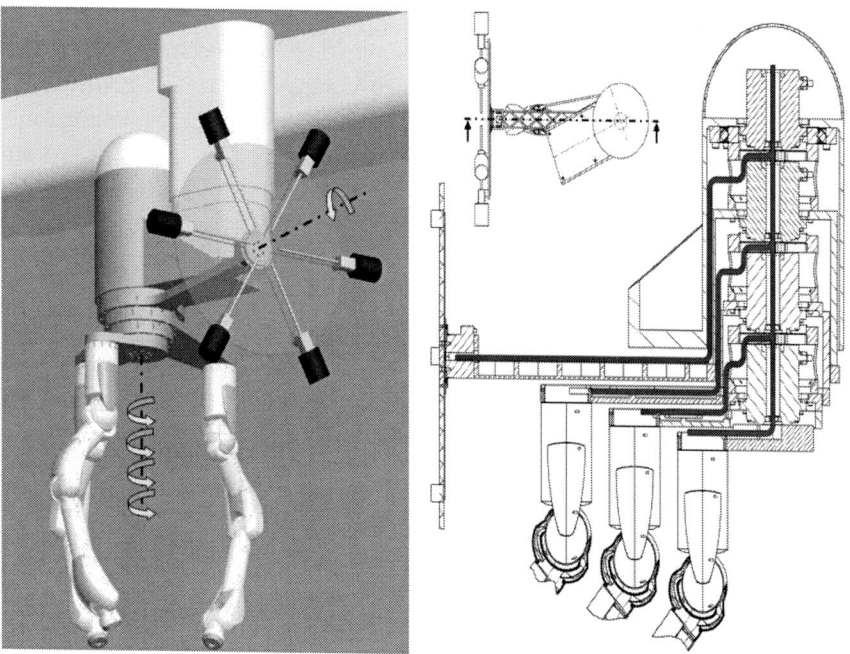

Figure 10. The CRHA carrying three DLR KineMedic® arms, and its cross-section view.

The CRHA ceiling mount is suggested common feature. The OR, will, then accommodate the combined CRHA/STAC equipment above the OT, in a space obstacle-free, not allowed to be crossed by the staff, when the robot is active. The general illumination panels can be arranged around the OT, not necessarily outside the robotic set-up. Checks of the light need to be performed, to insure that shadow areas are avoided and the required candlepower is guaranteed throughout the room.

To grant the required space to the anaesthetist, the robotic set-up is prevented from accessing to the area behind the patient's head. Only during neurosurgical operations, the robot is allowed to be located in the said space, kept otherwise by the anaesthetist. The monitors can be ceiling mounted, near the patient's feet. The other equipment, e.g. surgical lights and auxiliary ceiling mounted apparatus, should be arranged on both the sides of the patient, with the chance to slide on rails parallel to the OT. Adjustable booms allow the further regulation of the equipment. The proposed setup is supposed to optimise the OR workflow that varies with the pre-planning. It follows that, depending on the protocols, the robot workspace can be occupied either by the robotic system or by the staff.

The mini-probes carrier does not face pressing size constraints, chiefly, if the stiffness issue is guaranteed by active compensation. The considerably easier achievement, is balanced by the need of sustaining the mini probes coming out and precise insertion in the trocar opening. This, further exploits the "dispenser" back-castling, figure 8, where the mini-probes are packed.

Chapter 4

AUGMENTED REALITY ACTIONS

4.1. TASK-PLANNING OPERATION

The duty-split adds flexibility by versatility and redundancy. The **MIRS** objective, with resort to **CRHA** technology, addresses augmented intervention theatre, *IT*, exploiting complementary opportunities:

- computer integration, to enable transparent information framework, by enhanced monitoring and control aids;
- manipulation functional redundancy, to expand the effectors actions, by alternative intervention planning abilities.

The former opportunity has pace wise evolution, merging the ICT hardware/software innovations in the surgeons' habits, co-operatively showing the usefulness of the different programming functions. The latter one avails of the modularity of the **CRHA** mechanical architecture, carrying the KineMedic® arms, either the innovative mini-probes. The computer integration expands the intra-operative information flows, based on the pre-operation planning, initially pre-set by the surgeons, using the processed patient's images and the specific operation protocols. The expansion will progressively incorporate the **OR** data, possibly leading to **CRHA** and/or to **OT** up-dating.

With resort to duty-split, the information flow, figure 9, undergoes a series of steps, to plump for the govern mode: remote, autonomic or interactive, each time establishing what is under the surgeon either the assistant control/supervision. The idea is to alleviate the surgeon duty, conveying awareness to the assistant, notably, when the robot is not in contact with the patient. Besides, the task sequences requiring highest accuracy at the tiniest motion scale are, profitably, moved to the autonomic mode (and surgeon's supervision), again lowering the critical direct concern. An example suggestion leads to, figure 11:

- assistant duty allotment: **STAC** filling (step 1) and **CRHA** start-up/recovery command;
- surgeon duty allotment: patient registration (step 2) operation execution (step 6), after tool insertion and before tool withdrawal commands, up to abdomen deflation, trocars removal and incision suture (step 10);
- robot autonomic allotment: **CRHA** location (step 3), arms/instruments connection (step 4), instruments insertion (step 5), tools change (step 7), instrument withdrawal (step 8) and **CRHA** recovery (step 9).

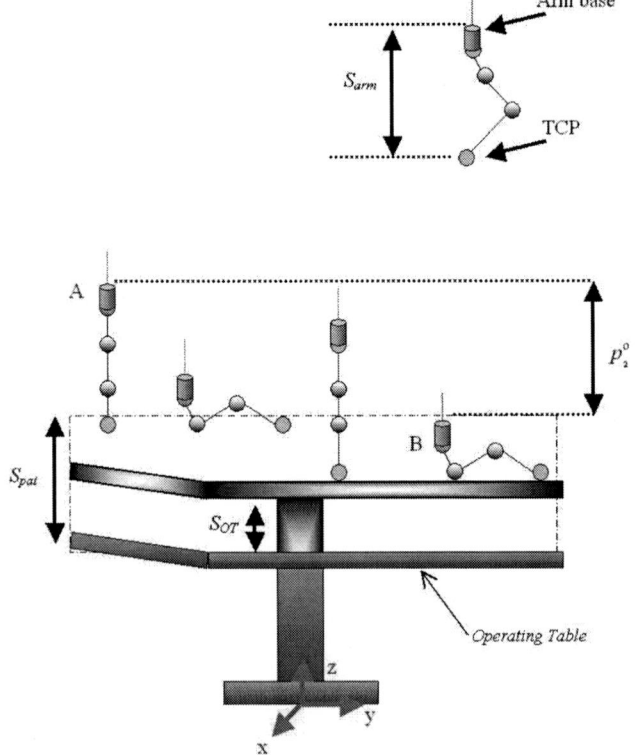

Figure 11. Parameters affecting the OT/CRHA coupling.

The suggested automatic steps can be done, for sure, under manual steering (of the surgeon/assistant). The **CRHA** location/recovery (steps 3/9) command can be done manually (mouse-driven). The arms/instruments connection (step 4), the insertion into and removal from the patient body (steps 5 and 8) and the tools change (step 7) procedures can be steered manually, whenever preferred. The suggested intra-operation schedule has the advantage to minimise relieve the surgeon duty; his panel is equipped with the commands allowing each time to control the individual devices, stopping the lower priority allotments.

The **CRHA** is deemed to become common complement in MIRS. Today, the DLR arms are dealt with as the standard reference, due to their modularity that assures easy integration. The LRP mini-probes are option to come, and are recalled to give explanatory hints by example arrangements, which, of course, lead to entirely different settings. For instance, when the **CRHA** vertical stroke, figure 11, is considered, the DLR arms can be located at a fixed height, in view of never working in fully stretched out configuration (near to the "elbow singularity"). The situation is considerably different with the LRP mini-probes; the co-operation environment might be necessary, with the concurrent vertical motion of the **CRHA**, of the operating table OT, or of both.

In both cases, the information flow avails of computer integration, notably, with resort to software aids (e.g., ambient-intelligence) and command/function redundancy. Both opportunities expand slowly, when one looks at actually running outfits.

4.2. INTELLIGENT PLANNING

The task agenda avails of graphical interfaces, for the surgeon and for the assistant, with ceiling mount, by resort to telescopic booms, to free the floor, figure 12. The latter shows the patient and robot (views from cameras at the **OR** ceiling corners); provides a list of statements, describing: the in-progress robot condition (e.g., tools in **STAC**), the safety margins (e.g., arms collision), the in-progress patient state (e.g., trocars inserted); and gives, by a colour code, the command state (ready, busy, fulfilled).

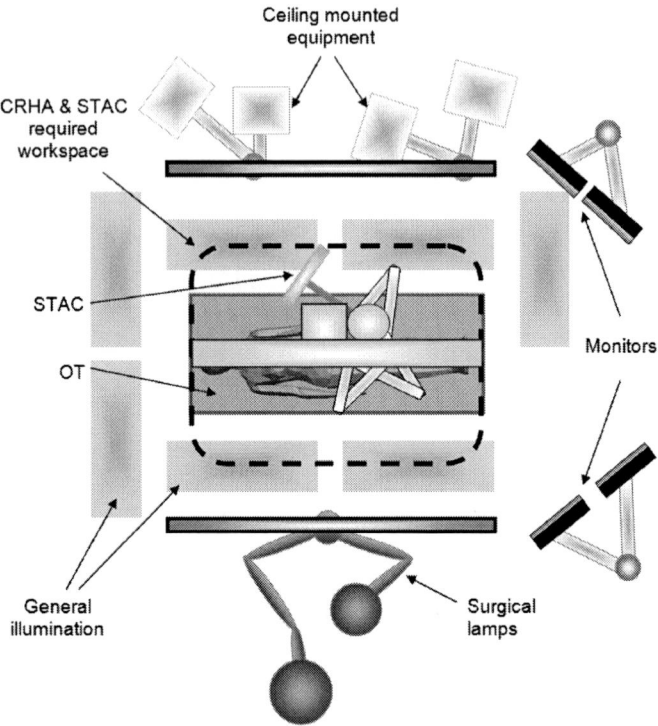

Figure 12. Ceiling set-up with included CRHA.

The **CRHA** ceiling mount is suggested common feature. The OR will, then, accommodate the combined **CRHA/STAC** equipment above the **OT**, in a space obstacle-free, not allowed to be crossed by the staff, when the robot is active. The general illumination panels can be arranged around the **OR**, close to the robotic set-up. Checks of the light need to be performed, to insure that shadow areas are avoided and the required candlepower is guaranteed throughout the room.

To grant the required space to the anaesthetist, the robotic set-up is prevented from accessing to the area behind the patient's head. Only during neurosurgical operations, the robot is allowed to be located in the said space, kept otherwise by the anaesthetist. The monitors can be ceiling mounted, near the patient's feet. The other equipment, e.g. surgical lights and auxiliary ceiling mounted apparatus, should be arranged on both the sides of the patient, with the chance to slide on rails parallel to the **OT**. Adjustable booms allow the further regulation of the equipment.

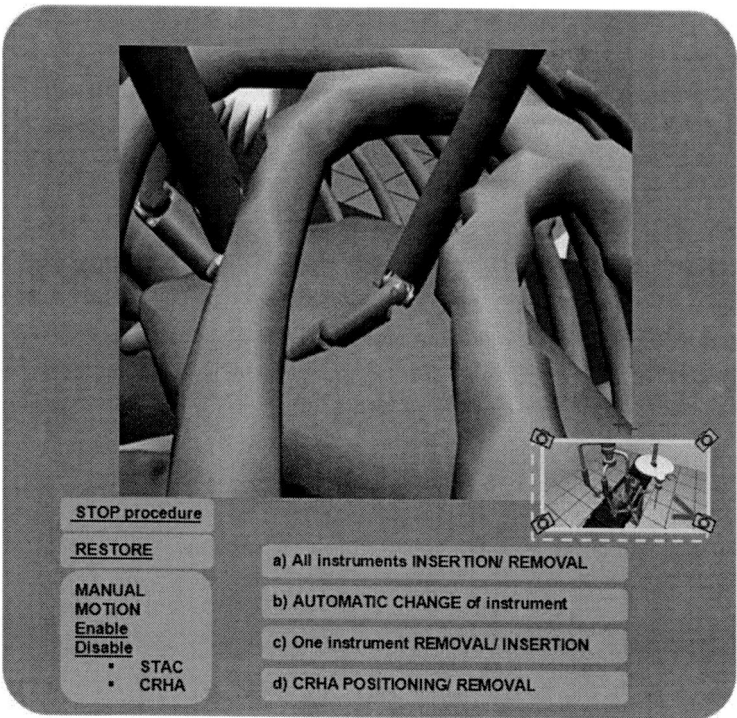

Figure 13. Example surgeon's monitor lay-out.

Exact functions are demanded to the surgeon's console (located with floor mount and ceiling connection to the hanging **CRHA**), which has to grant the precise control of the surgical instruments and of the endoscope, through reliable methods, intuitive procedures and ergonomic structures. The surgeon can switch to several windows; mainly, he focuses on 3D views in the intervention theatre, *IT*, selecting the desired zooming in or out, and enlarging or reducing the scene. Once the **CRHA** and robotic arms are in the planned positions to be introduced into the patient body, a green blinking signal on the top of the screen (the same that appears on the assistant's console) informs the surgeon that he/she can proceed, figure 13. The monitor bottom is equipped with keys; through them the automatic procedures are performed:

a) the instruments insertion and removal from the patient,
b) the automatic change of the instrument,
c) the removal and the insertion of one specific instrument,

d) the **CRHA** positioning and removal (same command as for the assistant).

When any of those orders is chosen, an extra window opens (on a side of the screen), where further options are given (like "insert" or "remove") and further selections are required; this reduces the risk that a procedure is involuntary executed. When, e.g., the change procedure (b) is selected, a guiding window opens, requiring the compulsory singling out of: the previous instrument; the new desired instrument; the key that initiates the change procedure. The third command (c) deals with removal and insertion of the selected instrument, but without including its change; it entails the opening of the guiding window, and could be needed, when an instrument has to be cleaned (e.g., the endoscope lens) or restored.

All the automatic procedures can be done only when certain requirements are fulfilled (e.g., the automatic **CRHA** positioning/removal (d) is authorised only if the instruments are outside the patient). The instruments are supposed to be controlled through two handles (for both left and right hand), positioned above the screen, to assure ergonomic workstation. Tremor suppression as well as force/haptic feedback are desirable options. The endoscope is supposed to be voice controlled (both for movement and zoom), with the intention to grant more freedom to the surgeon hands.

When an automatic procedure is carried out, a red blinking message on the centre top appears; at the same time, the handles are disabled preventing that remote-operation and automatic procedure coexist. Once this specific process ends, the message disappears and the surgeon can use the handles again to tele-operate. On the left bottom side of the screen, a set of *stop & start* keys allows to stop (or to restore) any automatic or remote-operated procedure; it provides the opportunity to switch to the manual control. On to the surgeon's requests, also the assistant's console can be similarly equipped. In case malfunction, a yellow blinking signal (on the screen left upper corner), alarms and informs the staff about the component and/or action failure. The interaction of handle and foot switches is, also, useful, to allow the surgeon not to leave/regain the handles at any choice. Further details are left out, to leave open to differently personalise the consoles.

To perform the quoted procedures, appropriate communication protocols need to establish among the system components. In that way, the server controls the procedures involved when accomplishing the intervention. The **CRHA** position, figure 14, or the **STAC** operation, figure 15, are example agendas detailed by the investigation.

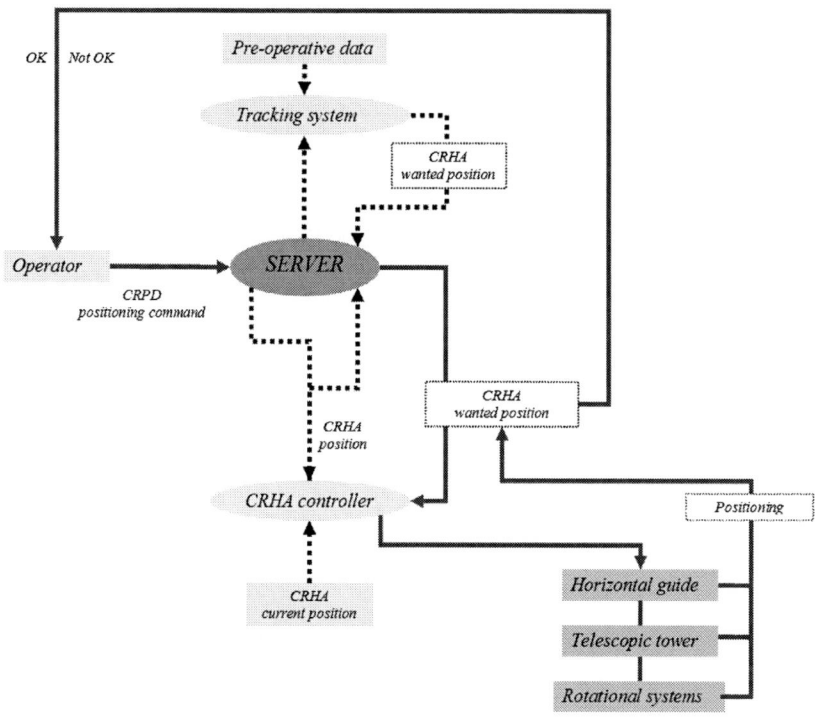

Figure 14. The CRHA positioning agenda.

In the second example, for instance, the procedure starts with the three operator's selections: the desired instrument, the previous instrument (which has to be replaced) and the command to start the procedure; these are sent to the main server. The server divides this data between the processor of the robotic arm (where the current instrument is attached) and the processor of the **STAC** (where the desired instrument is stored). The first step leads to the arm removal from the patient and to its positioning in the configuration planned for the instrument change. The server acts on the **STAC**, to allow it reaching the arm, and to provide an empty slot for the previous instrument; then, the action is repeated to fetch and to withdraw the new instrument. During the procedure, arm and **STAC** must know their relative position. For this reason, the data exchange leads every step and needs to be managed by the server. More sophisticated **STAC** are devised, to deal with the change of more instruments, through the simultaneous interaction with two or more arms.

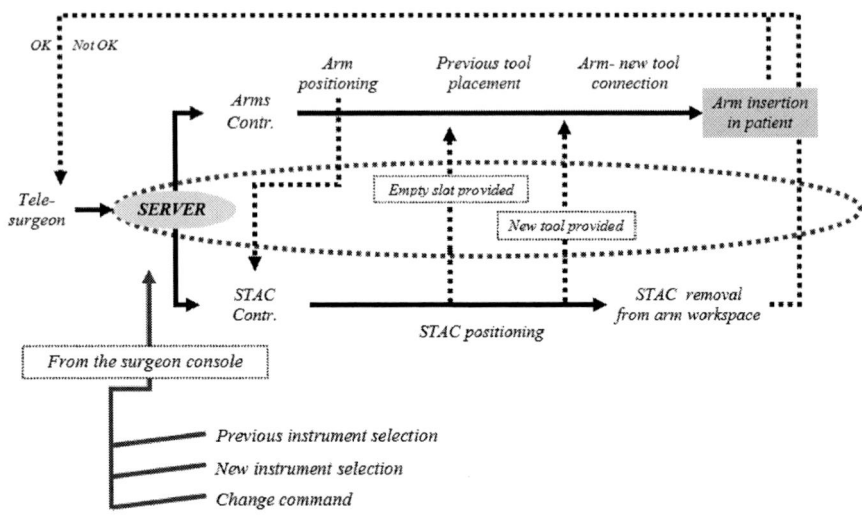

Figure 15. The STAC operation routine.

4.3. Emergency and Safety

The intra-operative communication is winning instrumental enabler in MIRS, and will become fundamental means to help exploit the robot functional redundancy, with time up-graded intervention protocols. The trend can be devised, firstly, looking at tasks management with today surgeon's (assistant's) consoles, figure 13, and following the duty-split prospects, when the (potentially) automatic procedures are performed. When any of above orders is chosen, an extra window opens (on the screen side), where the options appear (e.g., "insert", "remove", etc.) and further selection is required; this cuts the risk that any procedure is involuntary executed. When, e.g., the change procedure (b) is selected, the guiding window opens, compulsorily requiring to single out: the previous instrument; the new desired instrument; the key that initiates the change procedure. The third command (c) deals with removal/insertion of the selected instrument, but without its change; it entails the opening of the guiding window, and appears when it has to be cleaned (e.g., endoscope lens) or restored.

The front-end *IT* instrumentation becomes necessary aid. The automatic procedures can be done only when certain requirements are fulfilled (e.g., the automatic **CRHA** positioning/removal (d) is authorised only if the instruments are outside the patient). The instruments are supposed to be controlled through two handles (for both left and right hand), positioned above the screen, to assure ergonomic workstation. Tremor suppression as well as force/haptic feedback are desirable options. The endoscope is typically voice controlled (both for movement and zoom), with the intention to grant more freedom to the surgeon hands. When any automatic procedure is carried out, a red blinking massage on the centre top appears; at the same time, the handles are disabled preventing that remote-operation and automatic procedure coexist. Once this specific process ends, the message disappears and the surgeon can use the handles again to tele-operate. On the left bottom side of the screen, a set of *stop & start* keys allows to stop (or restore) any automatic or remote-operated procedure; it provides the opportunity to switch to the manual control. In case malfunction, a yellow blinking signal (on the screen left upper corner), alarms and informs about the component and/or action failure. The interaction of handle and foot switches permits the surgeon not to leave/regain the handles at any choice.

The discussed split-duty target is to improve the surgeon's ability by increasing his dexterity and accuracy, to obtain enhanced versatility and reliability, and, for the patient, better results in terms of higher efficiency and shorter hospitalisation. The robotic solution consistency is main aspect to assess, during its design. The bird-eye view on the study helps understanding that the **CRHA/STAC** addition fully complies every basic reliability and safety requests, at the present level of technologies (e.g., with resort to the DLR KineMedic® arms), and opens advanced prospects, when future nano-devices are made available (e.g. within the lines of the LRP mini-probe). A few remarks are summarised.

The need of highly safe procedures is especially important in the **OR** surroundings, where the robot has to interact with humans and equipment in constantly changing environment: in comparison to industrial robots, medical robotics is required to assist, rather then to replace the human work [Prouskas and Oakman, 2005; Speich and Rosen, 2004]. Even in the case of autonomous robots, the staff's presence is necessary during the setup of the equipment, as well as during the performance of the operation when the surgeon's supervision is required to monitor the correct advancement of the robot. This shows that *autonomic*, rather than *autonomous* behaviours, are addressed: the remote action is stepwise selected, monitored, controlled and up-dated by surgeon, and on-process robotic devices are only required to prosecute the pre-established task sequence, unless otherwise commanded. The all leads to safety charts that make the equipment reliable for the patient (and close surgical staff), figure 16, under constant overseeing.

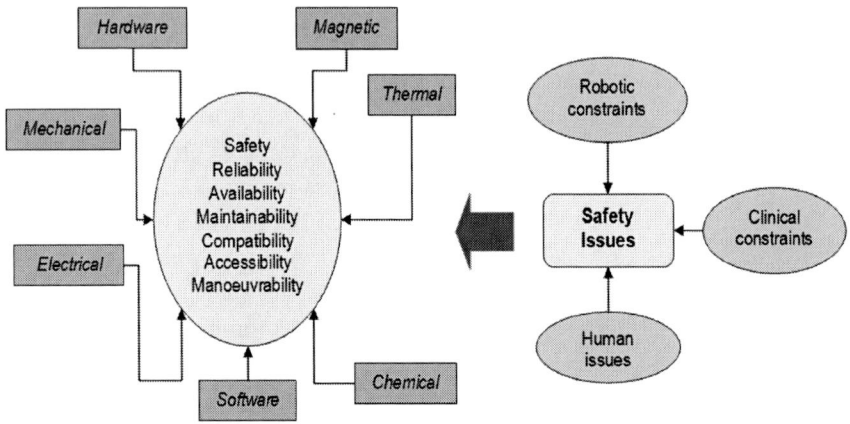

Figure 16. The safety opportunities.

The position accuracy is relevant feature. One needs to distinguish the **CRHA** pre-operative planned set-up that requires averaged figures, as tiny inaccuracies are trivial, due to, e.g., the registration process or patient motion (breathing, heart beating, etc.). The **CRHA** stiffness during the intervention is more critical: it can be achieved through posture monitoring and feedback compensation. Also, the redundancy in kinematics and encoders is common feature. Uncontrolled robot motion must be prevented, and sensors should be provided at the tool tip proximity, to avoid excessive forces on the patient that could result in involuntary dangerous damages of tissues. For that purpose, the patient's data registration is very helpful to establish the evolution of the procedure and the robot position according to the specific intervention.

Because unpredictable factors can occur (e.g., due to human errors, equipment malfunctions or unexpected patients complication), the pre-operative planning change must be possible, and intra-operative adjustments should be allowed, as well as fast removal of the robot from the patient. It is therefore important to provide manual manoeuvrability, either through back-drivable gears and, e.g., otherwise clutch systems. Moreover, the choice of motors determines the torque transmission and accuracy (harmonic drives or bevel gears could apply). Additionally, movements have to be limited to a well defined workspace, preserving patient and staff from potential collisions, but also preventing collisions inside the robot itself.

It is not only important to keep low the fault probability; it is also crucial to be capable to detect a potential fault and stop the system in time to avoid hazards. Redundant tele-operated and manually actuated parking brakes have to be available at emergency, including power break-down (fail safe). Easy manoeuvrability has to be taken in consideration, first, to make easy the surgeon's task, and second, to facilitate the access to the robot from the non clinical or technical staff (e.g. cleaning procedures).

The equipment availability and maintainability need to comply strict figures, with on-process diagnostics, proactive maintenance and ambient intelligence support. The accessibility to stop devices is granted by the keys duplication on the surgeon and on the assistant console. The control of the automatic procedures and of the manual settings is faced and implemented through intuitive interfaces. The equipment leanness is studied, to increase the availability and to assist the maintenance procedures. The proposed centralised control of the robotic system allows to isolate one or more desired components, without compromising the function of the remaining devices, leading to easier and faster inspections or repairs.

The choice to arrange the drives in serial vertical configuration (to grant the full 360° rotation to the arms) leads to increase the **CRHA** length. With the idea to lift the four drives on one side of the telescopic tower, providing cylindrical connectors to the arms connections, the **CRHA** withdrawal takes place granting free height of at least 2 m from the floor, optimising the space around the patient. The resort to optical fibre cables avoid the risk of electrocution [IEC 60601-1-2, 2007]. However, further analyses concerning the compatibility of the some details (e.g., the latch/unlatch **STAC** permanent magnets) have to be done, to avoid interferences with other **OR** equipment (e.g., defibrillators) or staff (e.g., personal belonging).

4.4. FUNCTIONAL REDUNDANCY

The split-duty approach, as it was pointed out at the beginning of the chapter, directly affects the backdrop aids (e.g., managing the end-effectors by co-robotic carriers and ambient intelligence tools); it, nevertheless, assures best performance through the synergic fusion with the forefront features (e.g., resorting to advanced equipment). To that purpose, the explanatory examples have addressed the DLR KineMedic® arms, to give a factual view of real implementations, and the LRP prototypal mini-probes, to deal with forefront features to come. In the chapter, task planning and manipulation agendas have given the thread to organise the concepts, along the complementary deployments: surgical planners, surgical effectors, surgical ambient-intelligence and surgical assistants. When dealing with robotic equipment, the man/machine interface, which assures the transfer of the surgeon expertise, know-how and proficiency, towards the MIRS intervention theatre, deserves the greatest relevance. To close the survey, a few comments on forefront features are given, sketching some side aspects, because, at the present state of the arts, are pioneering support (ambient-intelligence) and nice-implementation (robot with co-operation), and because, in the overall cutback, assures matching enablers.

Ambient intelligence, AmI; convergence of ubiquitous computing and ubiquitous communication, with duty-driven interfaces, adapting to the user. Three facts deserve explanation:

- ✓ **Ambient** – the concept assumes the ability of existing or be present on all sides
- ✓ **Ubiquitous** – it assumes that something exists everywhere, at the same time, on a steady level
- ✓ **Natural perception** – it involves self-adaptation, to match real life conditions.

The Ambient intelligence, AmI, incorporates properties of:

- ✓ **Mobile** (nomadic) computing, by multiple function devices and remote interaction capabilities
- ✓ **Distributed interactivity**, to enable communication by invisible processing computer resources
- ✓ **Self-adaptive multi-mode configuration**, to deal with the current human behavioral habits.

Ubiquitous computing is roughly the opposite of virtual reality. Where virtual reality puts people inside a computer-generated world, ubiquitous computing forces the equipment to operate in the real world, automatically adapting with the people preferences.

Figure 17. Ambient intelligence for real life monitoring.

The domain of ambient-intelligence, AmI, provides fast expanding tools to embed multi-media support in the man/machine interaction, figure 17. The AmI potentials are in the invisible backing of flexible and natural communication, with other users or computers, providing input and perceiving feedback, indifferently, with the resort to all senses and contact channels. The *ubiquitous computing* aims at invisibly and unobtrusively means, to free people from tedious routine jobs. In its final form, the concept leads to a computing device, which, when moving with the user, incrementally builds dynamic models of the changing environment and configures its services accordingly; it is able, either, to remember past patterns or proactively build up new ones [Michelini and Razzoli, 2007]. The *ubiquitous communication* is major change, promoting data transfer and allowing to integrate new modules, like sensors or diagnosis modules, by natural procedures [Gross and Fleisch, 2004].

The functional redundancy is basic idea in advanced robotics. The command redundancy is simple option, with different implementations, mainly, combining force and position feedbacks. The mobility redundancy is more complex setting, with several falls-off, exploring the combined co-operation of multiple-robot fixtures. The ability of separately closing position either force controls can be enabled for driving the robot to follow a trajectory, transmitting a pre-set effort law. During the robot work-phases, independent sensors provide the useful data for closing the appropriate feedback loops; when the state expansion makes possible to model the interfacing context, the dependence of force data and position data requires, either, the redundancy fading away (suppressing the over-specification), either, the extra data processing for calibration purposes.

The attribution of mobility redundancy is design trick to comply with, when the requested functions are not faced by six degrees-of-freedom. Mobility addition to an arm is good plot when, e.g., the effectors operate within a bounded work-space, before reached through a narrow entry; the trajectory and control planning, then, most of the times, divide in sub-tasks: approaching and operation. More specifically, the multi-robotic device appears innovation aiming at better reliability and/or effectiveness.

To assess the co-operation figures, the multi-functional framework specification is described, defining the relational structures of the task/performance cross-dependence and for the job-flow/resources concurrence. The co-operation problem is stated distinguishing control loops (closure of physical feedback) and decision schemes (closure of logic nets), to join the efficiency of the on-line command operation, with the flexibility of the on-process adaptivity, whenever requested by the application, figure 18. For the duty-specification, the aspects to investigate include:

- the function description of the agendas, to assess the advantages of robot co-operation;
- the execution constraints, with specification of the task programming requirements;
- the govern and information fit-out, to select the control and communication set-up.

Structures of the decision logic.	*hierarchic information tree-structure*: the co-operation among the robots is assured by a centralised control, under an explicitly established supervisor; *parallel-distributed information network*: to co-operation exists in a multi-agent cluster of units (sharing common interest data) interfaced through an intelligent layer.
Modes of the decision support.	to fulfil pre-scheduled steady operations, after command decentralisation; to perform job planning, re-setting the programmed-mode conditions; to recover the on-line control of the multi-robot facility, at emergencies.
Outputs of the govern module.	at the execution level, for enabling the operations of each individual robot; at the coordination level, for controlling the cooperation between robots; at the organisational level, for acknowledging the programmed tasks.

Figure 18. Decision-and-govern mode of co-operating robots.

Schedule meshing analysis, figure 19, is done at first, to recognise if duties are closely bounded, sequentially related or mainly self-sufficient; co-operation, in fact, increases operation efficiency, as robots share portions of the job, being able to perform a large variety of actions. The task complexity is, then, analysed, to set the handling architecture and to fix the govern level hierarchy, figure 20, namely:

- logic sequencing, at lower scheduler level, to comply with the nesting of (off-process specified) tasks "closed-duty" agendas, accomplishing in parallel prettily independent actions, to improve productivity;
- communicate-synchronise coordination, at intermediate planner level, to obtain the task-coordination by means of "sync-duty" operations, respecting the actions sequencing, with the priority constraints;
- decisional mechanisms activation, at upper controller level, for matching the tasks with the "open-duty" environment, in order to fulfil jobs actually requiring collaborative effort to grant reliable results.

CLOSED-DUTY	
The agendas are carried out simply managing the job parallelism.	
Several robots may operate in a given workspace, supervised by schedulers, with 'passive' constraints (e.g., for collision avoidance, etc.).	the decisional schemes are moved off-process; the command logic is pre-set, depending on execution stages ruled by the scheduler.
SYNC-DUTY	
The agendas are implemented exploiting appropriate functional sequencing.	
Planners govern the robots, with 'active' constraints on the job to be performed in parallel and/or in sequence.	the operation characterisation is detailed within the set of 'a priori' system-hypotheses; the task co-ordination follows a fixed logic, off-process assigned by (static) procedural knowledge.
OPEN-DUTY	
The agendas are built with procedural knowledge, shared by decentralised control units.	
Job progression is ruled by controllers, with embedded decisional aids that schedule the duty concurrence, based on the actual state updated information.	the robots functional characterisation is given, with the class of authorised tasks; the coordination is adapted, following to the on-process knowledge.

Figure 19. Scheduling by 'duty-mode' specification.

MANDATORY TASK CO-OPERATION	
Two or more robots, simultaneously or jointly, perform the job, with links on individual tasks such as:	
joint operated tasks	- the robots are doing a part of or the total job, for the fulfilment of which coupled co-operation is required.
simultaneous tasks	- the operations require more than one robot, e.g. one robot serves as a programmable fixture for other robots.
CONCURRENT TASK CO-OPERATION	
Two or more robots carry out, in parallel, portions of the same job, having independent charges such as:	
joint parallel tasks	- the robots work together on different facets of the same job, decreasing the total cycle time.
divide parallel tasks	- the robot diverse capabilities are exploited for specialised operations, e.g.: positioning, precision assembly, etc.
OPTIONAL TASK CO-OPERATION	
Any one of several robots can fulfil the all job, and only one is required, since the co-operation is based on:	
interchangeable tasks	- the responsibilities can dynamically be re-assigned among the robots, so that the job accomplishment is covered with failure backup.

Figure 20. Co-operation by 'task-mode' classification.

As third issue, the data sharing requests are considered, to be satisfied at:

- the (lower) operation range: scheduling/sequencing; devising/ planning; observing/controlling;
- the (upper) govern range: centralised (controller level) or decentralised (scheduler level) policy.

The design of efficient multi-robot equipment depends on the application. It can be viewed as the most satisfying set-up between conflicting goals, such as:

- duty flexibility *vs.* setting quickness;
- task versatility *vs.* job effectiveness;
- operation autonomy *vs.* quality assurance.

The solution choice needs to be explored at the design stage, referring to actual running conditions, to check functional and decisional options, exactly in the case duty-specification frame. The resort to digital mock-ups and virtual checks is handy means. Number of alternatives are explored, comparing charges and benefits and contrasting functional-to-decisional options, with quantitative figures of the robots performance.

The handling and govern structures are central issue to develop the fixture. The first characterises, defining the functional components: end-effectors, joints, kinematics chains, actuators, sensors, etc., and needs to be adapted to the manipulation requirement (i.e.: work-space, job requests, tasks agenda, information interfaces, control operations, etc.). Dexterity and accuracy push toward integrated sensing/command blocks and hybrid position/force control loops for the arms coordination. The govern structure, figure 18, has to adapt the actions to the current situations, related to on-going job-progression.

The preparation of the activity modes can be separated from their execution. The tasks given in charge to the co-robotic device, and the job fulfilment schedules (with related motion/wait conditions) are programmed (planner level) off-line; only the synchronisation is enabled during implementation. The co-operating robots govern, thus, requires an on-process communication structure between the units, figure 20, which assures:

- at the scheduler level, the monitoring of *closed-duty* agendas;
- at the planner level, the sequencing of *sync-duty* agendas;
- at the controller level, the coordination of *open-duty* agendas.

The scheduler activates the tasks parallelism, once verified the requested job sequencing. The controller, congruent with flexible surroundings, requires the full visibility on tasks progression, to exploit the updated knowledge on current situations, to modify the agenda, depending on the scheduled duties and, eventually, to adapt the robot behaviour in relation to the situational changes. The context brings to a hierarchic knowledge reference frame, to distinguish the 'external' from the 'internal' structural conditions and to prepare solving procedures, consistent with the acknowledged relational schemes. The planner, in-between, is specifically addressed by the duty-split approach, at least at the present state of arts, when the **CRHA** implement assures the mentioned task-planning prospects, since the agendas are ran using embedded functional sequencing. The limited thrust/torque capability of future micro-effectors might require to turn to more sophisticated **CRHA** agendas; the controller level could represent better solution, with the co-operation enabled by the procedural knowledge, in common between distributed processing blocks.

Chapter 5

CONCLUSION

5.1. THE REFERENCE DEVELOPMENTS

The robotic surgery is already at advanced level, with sophisticated implementations covering the many areas where the high accuracy, the tremor filtering, the force control, the radiation protection, etc. suggest the interposition of a slave actuation, assuring the enhanced effectiveness and reliability to the remote handling under the surgeon's control. The master/slave setting is, perhaps, unconscious answer of the anthropocentric approaches; it is not the most task-suited or operator-friendly. The one-to-one motion/force duplication is, by now, already over-rid by the present robotic augmentation, assuring the information widening by haptic links and duty efficiency by miniaturised probes. The development of strictly task-driven equipment can profit by that, aiming at the conceiving purposely designed devices, for every specific application, more or less, as the fixed-automation fixtures assured the most effective answer to the earlier manufacturing facilities. The lack of flexibility could be severe hindrance, when the actual intervention has to face unexpected occurrences, so that robotics should be exploited in terms of the surroundings intelligence and autonomy management, more than in terms of task programming and function bent capabilities. The microsurgery robotic augmentation is, thereafter, appearing as the challenge for enhanced solutions, along the lines of the instrumental robotics.

5.2. THE PROSPECTED ARCHITECTURE

The MIRS perspectives will totally modify the way the surgeons deal with in-body operations. Today, the technique sophistication, typically, moves along anthropocentric tracks, when the intervention theatre needs to be reached by hand-carried tools and shall grant direct visual observation. Robotic surgery opens wholly different options, but noteworthy outcomes do not suffer only technology gaps, as, first of all, sophistication should encompass relevant paradigm shifts in the operation protocols. This means rather altered approaches in the design of the robotic instrumental aids; therefore, the present investigation has faced notable issues, combining the minimally invasive robotic surgery technique with the duty-split idea [Michelini and Razzoli, 2008]. For concreteness, the research preferred continuous feasibility checks, thus, the co-robotic means and planning deal with existing developments: the high performance modular DLR arms and the (some slightly futuristic) miniature probes. This way, both, actual and on-progress options are considered, bringing forward the procedural innovation as preliminary step of the instrumental up-dating.

On these assumptions, the functional versatility of the co-robotic equipment ought to be explored, linked to the capabilities of the front effectors. The enhanced performance can be enabled on-progress, depending on the articulated probe/arm advances. Typically, for instance, the constraint on mobility aims at making given achievements feasible, disregarding the (more or less relevant) side-effects. Invasiveness is lowered, but not avoided, when vital organs are involved. Now, an articulated in-body probe has better dexterity with blocks higher in number and smaller in size; cable-actuation quickly faces unavoidable drawbacks, due to the force-coupling among blocks. Happily, the current micro-electro-mechanical-systems, **mems**, technology provides effective means to obtain proper arrangements, and future devices will, most likely, quickly assure improved performance. In any case, the duty-split idea permits conceiving auxiliary carriers fitted out for evolving end-effectors, as soon as these are made available.

This suggests the parallel investigation of both reference technologies. An advanced auxiliary carrier, the **CRHA**, is presented in this study. A thorough analysis of current situations in the OR suggests to dispose of a considerable level of automation, enabling the accurate arm positioning.

Conclusion 45

The co-robotic equipment, this way, integrates seamlessly into the surgical workflow. The prospected operative agendas already undertake duties out of standard man reach, however, fully maintaining standard habits in problem solving. To that view, the analysis addresses four complementary deployments: surgical planners, surgical effectors, surgical ambient-intelligence and surgical assistants, each time singling out, rather than technology-driven solutions, factual opportunities to deal with acknowledged actions of the current interventional medicine.

This way, «computer integration», simply, presents as "augmented reality" opportunity, to quite naturally enhance the man capabilities, not only by special-purpose operating tools, but, as well, by supporting frames and information handlers. The computer-aided surgery will become routine technique, covering synergistic areas: modelling and analysis of patients and surgical sequences, instrumental end-effectors, man-machine interface technology, and systems science for equipment/protocol safety and reliability. The robotic surgery develops to work out duty-driven implements, based on domain knowledge and expertise. The state of arts in the four areas is quickly evolving, and this affects the actual achievements, with relevant steps ahead as soon as the appropriation of a new technology makes it possible exploring more advanced issues. For instance, in the man-machine interface, 'the ambient intelligence' could appear limited and static option; the approach is deemed to open dynamic effects, to the advantage of the overall interfacing infrastructure, warranting higher performance, with immediately perceived falls-off in the other three areas.

Similarly, at the present technological stage, the **CRHA/STAC** proposal permits to manage the functional redundancy by, basically, "sync-duty" schedules, figure 19. The duty-split approach, thereafter, is implemented to follow appropriate functional sequencing, where the intermediate targets check provides factual benefits in terms of effectiveness and reliability. The 'static' option is limited improvement, as similar achievements are already provided by resorting, e.g., to the DLR arms directly positioned, without co-operating carrier. The all progressively modifies, if the duty-split is interpreted dynamically, with the leeway of schedules reallocation. This requires combining the foreground knowledge: pre-operative (modelling, simulation and planning) and intra-operative (process overseeing and execution helps), with the background knowledge: domain (surgery expertise) and ancillary (actuators, sensors and information handling instrumentation). The issues shall face the decision-and-govern mode prospects, figure 18, and enable operative schedules, with on-process account of the functional redundancy.

The 'dynamic' option, in the said context, represents the evolution of the computer-aided surgery towards integrated solutions, embedding the mentioned four synergistic areas. Pace-wise progression is expected to follow, due to the peculiarity, in terms of safety and reliability, of interventions on the human body under the surgeon's responsibility. The robotic equipment, having human multifarious abilities, does not get the whole or share a part of responsibility; this means that the master/slave concept remains the only valid paradigm in the domain, even when, once the technologies appropriation is completed, the automatic management of the functional versatility brings in precious rewards. We face the subtle condition, where minimal invasiveness means to go below the resolution of the human sensorial capabilities, while the intervention credibility and consistency is instigated at the anthropic scale. At the moment, the research outcomes meet with light and shadow: thriving successes (e.g., endoscope's 3D video-restitution by controlled image magnification) and deceptive limitations (e.g., the thrust/torque want of existing nano-effectors); besides, we keep on with the customary diagnoses and treatments habits, highly affected by traditional medical patterns.

5.3. FUTURE WORK AND CONCLUSION

Surgery requires high trustworthiness and reliability, and only fully tested and safe devices are deemed to be taken into account. The duty-split approach, nonetheless, addresses the handling architecture of advanced robotic surgical planners, aiming at widening the function versatility by background potential, while leaving the pace-wise technological up-turning to the foreground additions, each time, if the proper confidence is attained. Clearly human reasoning should never be replaced completely by robots, and this design principle is especially crucial in surgical robotics. The ideas shown in this work, therefore, follow the approach of the "best-of-skill" co-operation, figure 21, combining the strengths of the human mastery, the robotic reliance and the ambient intelligence. The surgeon is in control of the whole procedure in all times, with non critical tasks entrusted to autonomic robot capabilities and to exhaustive knowledge-management aids.

The split-duty approach in robotic surgery, according to the out-lined considerations, appears to be notably useful to deal with computer integrated opportunities. When the **CRHA** equipment is used for managing the base positioning of assessed-technology manipulation arms, such as the DLR KineMedic®, the steps into the integration remain at comparatively shallow depth. Technical considerations, such as the optimal robot base positioning are handled by the pre-operative planner, whereas the surgeon can fully concentrate on working with the special-purpose effectors in optimal performance configuration, automatically managed by the main processor. Considerations to further enhance the surgical procedure directly lead to the idea of the automatic changing device for surgical tools, **STAC**. The design of such a fixture falls in the scopes of this work, and this was shown to be basically possible, although with cautions, when the sterility of unused tools has to be maintained. The further development of automatic devices, to timely equip the robot with the required tools, is, undoubtedly, a seminal research direction. In a long term view, the entire circulation of sterilised tools has to be made automatic, enabling autonomous handling, logistics, treatment and delivery, leaving to the surgeon (and/or to the assistant) the basic charge of overseeing and controlling.

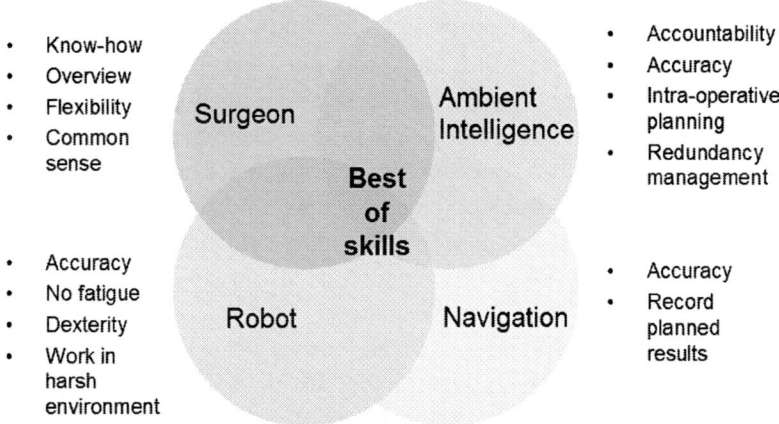

Figure 21. Man/robot co-operation by "best-of-skill" concept.

Within the duty-split philosophy, the operation mode, basically, draws near the 'closed-duty', figure 19, with no sophisticated co-operation requirements. When the **CRHA** equipment is used for managing the support of advanced-technology manipulation devices, such as the LRP mini-probes, considerably more complex help is needed. The articulated probe is assumed to approach the intervention theatre with 'optimal' attitude of the front tip, after 'optimal' trajectories, duly avoiding every sensible organ. The rank 'optimal' is established at pre-operative planning, but, certainly, corresponds to time-varying settings along with the intervention, even if fully self-

exhaustive patients models and surgical sequences are established. With the duty-split approach, the operation mode, typically, turns to the 'open-duty', figure 19, specification, requiring on-process variation. The nice conduct of the task-planning prospects cannot, anymore, bring to simple information flows, as the local situations are brought forth with interlaced chains.

The paradigm shift in the duty-split approach leads to managing the functional redundancy by intervention fusion methods and tools. When dealing with future prospects, these methods and tools are crucial challenge, and need to be warily accounted for to devise the robotic surgery to come. In the present survey, an example **CRHA** equipment for the LRP mini-probes is out-lined, simply, to show the feasibility and to evidence some peculiarities. For instance, the probe compliance and looseness make difficult the firm deployment of current modules; the 'dispenser' storing and guide might represent worthy contrivance, provided that the trocar entry task is simultaneously steered; the all, very soon, becomes 'open-duty' agenda, calling decision-and-govern protocols. The study of such protocols falls beyond the scopes of this work, and is omitted, because the mini-probe, at its prototypal state, cannot be used for a deeper investigation.

All in all, however, the survey cannot neglect providing the sketches of future scenarios, not only as guess of futuristic outcomes, rather also as factual indication of practical means and implements. This suggests to tackle the robotic surgery, within the framework of the duty-split approach, looking, first of all, at the trends towards computer-aided surgery as self-consistent objective, requiring four complementary deployments, to deal with technology-driven instruments, which, nevertheless, need to reach appropriateness, due to the inner peculiarity, as for safety and reliability. The conceptual design of the **CRHA** equipment, thereafter, permits to make a survey, where technologies have the instrumental role they deserve, in front of the supplied problem-solving potential. The focus on the duty-split philosophy moves accordingly; it brings insight on innovative prospects, by out-lining their methodological support. The question is not to invent a technical answer for an, up-now, unsolved problem; rather, to devise alternative instruments and protocols that could represent more effective ways out. Moreover, the decision about the alternatives is totally left to the surgeon, who bears the whole responsibility of the intervention and should feel fully confident on technologies and methodologies.

REFERENCES

Antypas, C., and Pantelis, E. (2008) Performance evaluation of a CyberKnife® G4 image-guided robotic stereotactic radiosurgery system. *Phys. Med. Biol., vol. 53*, pp. 4697-4718.

Bidaud, P. Sallé, D., and Cepolina, F. (2004).Task based optimization method for the design of modular minimally invasive surgery instruments. *15th CISM-IFToMM Symposium on Robot Design, Dynamics and Control*, Montreal, Canada.

Cepolina, F. (2005). Development of micro-tools for surgical applications. *Ph.D. Thesis*, Università di Genova, Italy & Université P. & M. Curie, Paris.

Cepolina, F., and Michelini R.C. (2003). A family of co-robotic surgical set-ups. *Intl. J. Industrial Robots, vol. 30, no. 6*, pp. 564-574.

Cepolina, F., and Michelini, R.C. (2005). Trends in robotic surgery. *Intl. J. Recent Advances in Urology, vol. 19, no. 8*, pp. 940-951.

Cepolina, F., Michelini, R.C. (2004). Review of robotic fixtures for minimal invasive surgery. *Intl. J. Medical Robotics & Computer-Assisted Surgery, vol. 1, no. 1*, pp. 43-63.

Damiano, R.J., Ehrman, W.J., Ducko, C.T., et al. (2000). Initial Unite States clinical trial of robotically assisted coronary artery bypass grafting. *J. Thorac. Cardiovasc. Surg., vol. 119*, pp. 77-82.

Detter, C., Deuse, T., Christ, F., Boehm, D.H., Reichenspurner, H., Reichart, B. (2002). Comparison of two stabilizer concepts for offpump coronary artery bypass grafting. *Ann. Thorac. Sur., vol. 74*, pp. 497-501.

Farokhzad, O.C., and Langer R, (2006). Nano-medicine: developing smarter therapeutic and diagnostic modalities. *Adv. Drug Deliv. Rev., vol. 58, no. 14*, pp. 1456-1459.

Fine, H., Wei, W., Chang, S., Simaan, N. (2009). A novel dual-arm dexterous ophthalmic microsurgical robot: applications for retinal vascular cannulation and stent deployment. *American Society of Retinal Specialists, Retina Congress*, New York, NY.
Frumento, S. (2006). Design of co-robotic devices for minimally invasive robotic surgery. *Ph.D. Thesis*, PMAR Lab, University of Genova, Italy.
Frumento, S., Michelini, R.C., Konietschke, R., Hagn, U., Ortmaier, T., and Hirzinger, G. (2006). A co-robotic positioning device for carrying surgical end-effectors. *Proc. of Intl. Conf. ASME-ESDA*, Torino, July 4-7, pp.1-8.
Gross, S., and Fleisch, E. (2004). Maintenance improvement by unique product information enabled by ubiquitous computing. *Proc. of 11th Intl. IFAC Symp. Information Control Problems in Manufacturing*, Salvador, Brasil, pp. 65-70.
Guerrouad, A., and Vidal, P. (1989). S.M.O.S.: Stereotaxical Microtelemanipulator for Ocular Surgery. *Proc. Annual Int. Conf. IEEE Engineering in Medicine and Biology Society*, vol. 11, pp. 879-880.
Guthart, G. and Salisbury, K. (2000). The intuitiveTM telesurgery system: overview and application. *Proc. of 2000 IEEE International Conference on Robotics and Automation*, pp. 618-621.
Hashizume, M., and Tsugawa, K., (2004). Robotic Surgery and Cancer: the Present State, Problems and Future Vision. *Japanese Journal of Clinical Oncology*, vol. 34, pp. 227-237.
IEC 60601-1-2 (Ed.3.0). (2007). *Medical electrical equipment - Part 1-2: General requirements for basic safety and essential performance - Collateral standard: Electromagnetic compatibility - Requirements and tests.*
Intuitive Surgical. (2006). *Company Profile - Investor Relations FAQ*. http://www.intuitivesurgical.com/.
Jacobs, S., Holzhey, D., Kiaii, B.B., Onnasch, J.F., Walther, T., Mohr, F.W., and Falk, V. (2003). Limitations for manual and telemanipulator-assisted motion tracking—implications for endoscopic beating-heart surgery. *Ann. Thorac. Surg.*, vol. 76, pp. 2029-2035.
Konietschke, R., Weiß, H., Ortmaier, T., and Hirzinger, G. (2004). A preoperative planning procedure for robotically assisted minimally invasive interventions. *Jahrestagung der Deutschen Gesellschaft fur Computer-und Roboterassistierte Chirurgie*, (Muenchen, Germany), pp.1-6.
Kumar, R., Berkelmen, P., Gupta P., Barnes, A., Jensen, P., Whitcomb, L., and Taylor, R.H. (2000). Preliminary experiments in cooperative human/robot

force control for robot assisted microsurgical manipulation. *Proceedings of ICRA*, pp- 610-617.

Lum, M.J.H., Trimble, D., Rosen, J., Fodero II, K., King, H., Sankarayanaranan, G., Dosher, J., Leushke, R., Martin-Anderson, B., Sinanan, M.N., and Hannaford, B. (2006). Multidisciplinary approach for developing a new minimally invasive surgical robot system. *Proceedings of the 2006 BioRob Conference*, Pisa, Italy, pp. 841-846.

Michelini, R.C., Razzoli, R.P. (2007). Ubiquitous computing & communication for product monitoring. In Khosrow-Pour, M. (Ed.). *Encyclopaedia of Information Science and Technology* (2nd edition, pp. 3851-3857), Hershey, PA: Idea Group Inc.

Michelini, R.C., Razzoli, R.P. (2008). Co-operative minimally invasive robotic surgery. *Industrial Robot, vol. 35, no. 4*, pp. 347-360.

Miroir, M., Szewczyk, J., Nguyen, Y., Mazalaigue, S., Bozorg Grayeli, A., and Sterkers, O. (2008). Mechanical Design and Optimization of a Microsurgical Robot. *Proceedings of EUCOMES*, Springer, Netherlands, pp. 575-583.

Prouskas, C.B., and Oakman, A. (2005). *Medical robotics survey.* http://www.doc.ic.ac.uk/~nd/surprise_96/journal/vol4/ao2/report.html

Reintsema, D., Ortmaier,T., Preusche, C., Hirzinger, G. (2004). Toward High-Fidelity Telepresence in Space and Surgery Robotics. *Presence, vol. 13, no. 1*, pp. 77-98.

Rosen, J., and Hannaford, B. (2006). Doc at a distance: robot surgeons promise to save lives in remote communities, war zones, and disaster-stricken areas. *IEEE Spectrum, vol. 42, no. 10*, pp. 34-39.

Sallé, D., Cepolina, F., and Bidaud, P. (2004). Surgery grippers for minimally invasive heart surgery. *Proc. of IEEE International Conference on Intelligent Manipulation and Grasping IMG 04*, Genova, Italy, pp. 1-8.

Seibold, U., Kubler, B., and Hirzinger, G. (2005). Prototype of instrument for minimally invasive surgery with 6-axis force sensing capability. *Proceedings of the 2005 IEEE International Conference on Robotics and Automation ICRA*, (Barcelona, Spain), pp. 498-503.

Silva, G.A. (2007). Nanotechnology approaches for drug and small molecule delivery across the blood brain barrier", *Surg. Neurol., vol. 67, no. 2*, pp.113-116.

Speich, J.E.. and Rosen, J. (2004). Medical robotics. In: Wnek, G. and Bowlin, G. (Eds.). *Encyclopaedia of Biomaterials and Biomedical Engineering* (pp. 983-993). New York, NY: Marcel Dekker.

Taylor, R.H., Jensen, M., Whitcomb, L., et al. (1999). A steady-hand robotic system for microsurgical augmentation. *Robot Res., vol. 12*, pp. 1201-1210.

Wei, W., Ku, K., Simaan, N. (2006). A Compact Two-Armed Slave Manipulator for Minimally Invasive Surgery of the Throat. *The first IEEE/RAS-EMB International Conference on Biomedical Robotics and Biomechatronics*, Pisa, Italy, pp. 287-292.

INDEX

A

abdomen, 26
accuracy, 1, 2, 7, 17, 18, 26, 33, 34, 40, 43
achievement, 24
activation, 38
actuation, 6, 8, 19, 43, 44
actuators, 5, 40, 45
alternative, 8, 25, 48
anatomy, 6
anterior cruciate, 12
anthropic, 46
application, 37, 40, 43, 50
artery, 10, 49
assumptions, 44
attribution, 37
automation, 7, 43, 44
autonomous robot, 33
autonomy, 40, 43
availability, 35
avoidance, 39
awareness, 25

B

back, 7, 24, 34
benefits, 17, 40, 45
blocks, 40, 41, 44
blood, 1, 51
booms, 24, 27, 28
brain, 14, 15, 51
brain structure, 14
breathing, 34
bypass, 49

C

cables, 35
calibration, 37
carrier, 23, 24, 44, 45
catheter, 5, 9
cerebrospinal fluid, 1
changing environment, 33, 36
circulation, 47
CISM, 49
classification, 39
clinical trial, 49
collaboration, 9
collision avoidance, 39
collisions, 34
communication, 30, 32, 36, 37, 40, 51
compatibility, 35, 50
compensation, 24, 34
complementarity, 18
complexity, 1, 8, 38
compliance, 48

complications, vii, ix, 10, 21
components, 18, 30, 35, 40
computing, 36, 50, 51
configuration, 7, 27, 31, 35, 47
constraints, 6, 24, 37, 38, 39
control, x, 1, 2, 6, 9, 10, 14, 18, 19, 21, 25, 27, 29, 30, 33, 35, 37, 38, 39, 40, 43, 46, 51
coronary artery bypass graft, 49
coupling, 26, 44
covering, 43, 45
credibility, 46

D

data processing, 37
data transfer, 36
decentralisation, 38
definition, 19
deflation, 26
disabled, 30, 33
duplication, 35, 43

E

elbow, 27
endoscope, 2, 5, 6, 29, 30, 32, 33, 46
endoscopy, 14
environment, 27, 38
evolution, 1, 18, 25, 34, 46
execution, 2, 17, 26, 37, 38, 39, 40, 45
expertise, 3, 18, 19, 36, 45
exposure, 10
eye, 6, 9, 17, 33

F

feedback, 7, 30, 33, 34, 36, 37
feeding, 19
feet, 24, 28
flexibility, ix, 6, 17, 25, 37, 40, 43
flow, 25, 27, 37
fluid, 1

Food and Drug Administration (FDA), 10, 14
fusion, 35, 48

G

grafting, 49
groups, 6, 7

H

hands, 10, 30, 33
haptic, ix, 6, 7, 30, 33, 43
hazards, 35
heart, 10, 34, 50, 51
height, 20, 27, 35
hip, 10, 11, 12
hip replacement, 10, 11, 12
hospital, ix
hospitals, vii, 10
human, x, 1, 2, 3, 6, 8, 9, 10, 17, 18, 33, 34, 46, 50
humans, 33

I

ICT, 2, 25
illumination, 23, 28
images, 5, 7, 25
immersion, 19
implementation, 35, 37, 40, 43
in situ, 6, 21
indication, 48
industrial, 7, 20, 33
industrial application, 7
infrastructure, 2, 17, 45
innovation, 18, 21, 37, 44
insertion, 5, 21, 24, 26, 27, 29, 30, 32
insight, 7, 48
inspections, 35
instruments, 6, 7, 26, 27, 29, 30, 31, 32, 48, 49
integration, 2, 3, 18, 25, 27, 45, 46

intelligence, ix, 1, 3, 5, 7, 8, 18, 19, 27, 35, 36, 43, 45, 46
interaction, 30, 31, 33, 36
interface, 3, 5, 36, 45
interference, 6
intermediate targets, 45
intervention, ix, x, 1, 3, 5, 6, 7, 8, 17, 18, 19, 21, 25, 29, 30, 32, 34, 36, 43, 44, 46, 47, 48
invasive, vii, ix, x, 1, 3, 5, 9, 18, 44, 49, 50, 51

J

jobs, 36, 38
joints, 8, 40

K

kinematics, 34, 40
knee, 7, 10, 12
knee replacement, 10, 12

L

laparoscope, 13
laparoscopic, 9, 13
laparoscopic surgery, 13
lens, 30, 32
ligament, 12
limitations, 8, 17, 46
linear, 13, 20
linkage, 13
links, 39, 43
liquidation, 12
localised, 2
location, 6, 7, 11, 20, 21, 26, 27
logistics, 47

M

M.O., 50
magnets, 35

maintenance, 35, 50
management, 1, 32, 43, 46
manipulation, ix, 2, 5, 6, 7, 9, 13, 19, 25, 35, 40, 46, 47, 51
manufacturing, 43
mastery, 8, 46
medicine, 2, 3, 45, 49
microsurgery, 1, 6, 43
mobility, 19, 23, 37, 44
modalities, 49
models, 2, 36, 48
modules, 36, 48
motion, 2, 6, 7, 9, 26, 27, 34, 40, 43, 50
motors, 13, 34
mouse, 27
mouth, 2
movement, 30, 33

N

natural, 2, 7, 9, 36
network, 38
neurosurgery, 1

O

oncology, 50
operator, 6, 31, 43
ophthalmic, 6, 50
optical, 35
optimal performance, 47
optimization, 2, 49
optimization method, 49
organ, 20, 47
orthopaedic, 10
oversight, 1

P

paradigm shift, 44, 48
parallelism, 39, 41
passive, 6, 7, 8, 17, 39
patients, 13, 14, 18, 34, 45, 48
perception, 7

philosophy, 18, 47, 48
physiological, 6
planning, 2, 6, 14, 18, 19, 21, 24, 25, 34, 35, 37, 38, 40, 41, 44, 45, 47, 50
plastic, 14
posture, 8, 34
power, 35
pre-planning, 24
proactive, 35
probability, 35
probe, 20, 21, 33, 44, 47, 48
problem solving, 45
problem-solving, 48
procedural knowledge, 39, 41
productivity, 38
profit, 43
programming, 1, 19, 25, 37, 43
property, iv
protection, 43
protocol, 45
protocols, ix, 1, 2, 5, 6, 8, 19, 23, 24, 25, 30, 32, 44, 48
prototype, 7

Q

quality assurance, 40

R

radiation, 10, 43
range, 2, 6, 7, 9, 13, 40
RAS, 52
reconstruction, 12
recovery, 19, 26, 27
redundancy, 8, 19, 25, 27, 32, 34, 37, 45, 48
reference frame, 41
regulation, 24, 28
relevance, 36
reliability, 17, 18, 19, 33, 37, 43, 45, 46, 48
resolution, 46
resources, 37
responsibilities, 39
restitution, 17, 46

retina, 6
rewards, 46
risk, 30, 32, 35
robotic, vii, ix, x, 2, 6, 7, 8, 9, 10, 18, 19, 20, 23, 28, 29, 31, 33, 35, 37, 40, 43, 44, 45, 46, 48, 49, 50, 51, 52
robotic arm, 20, 29, 31
robotic surgery, x, 43, 44, 45, 46, 48, 49, 50, 51
robotics, vii, ix, 1, 2, 17, 18, 33, 37, 43, 46, 49, 50, 51, 52

S

safety, 1, 14, 17, 27, 33, 34, 45, 46, 48, 50
scaling, 7
scheduling, 40
selecting, 29
sensing, 6, 40, 51
sensitivity, 18
sensors, 5, 19, 34, 36, 37, 40, 45
sequencing, 38, 39, 40, 41, 45
sharing, 38, 40
signals, 15
simulation, 45
sites, 1, 5
skills, x, 9
software, 18, 25, 27
stability, 9
stent, 50
stiffness, 24, 34
strategies, 17, 19, 21
stroke, 27
strokes, 20
supervision, 2, 3, 25, 33
supervisor, 38
suppression, 30, 33
surgeons, 2, 3, 18, 25, 44, 51
surgeries, 14
surgery, vii, ix, x, 1, 2, 3, 5, 6, 7, 9, 10, 11, 13, 14, 15, 17, 18, 19, 21, 43, 44, 45, 46, 48, 49, 50, 51, 52
surgical, vii, ix, x, 2, 3, 6, 8, 10, 13, 15, 17, 18, 19, 23, 24, 28, 29, 34, 36, 45, 46, 47, 48, 49, 50, 51

surgical intervention, 2, 19
suture, 26
switching, 21
synergistic, 45, 46

U

ultrasound, 14
user-defined, 14

T

technological developments, 5
technology gap, 44
torque, 34, 41, 46
training, 9
trajectory, 37
transfer, 3, 36
transmission, 2, 34
transparency, 18
transparent, 25
tremor, 6, 43
trial, 49
trustworthiness, 19, 46

V

validation, 2
variation, 48
versatility, ix, 6, 17, 18, 25, 33, 40, 44, 46
visualization, 9
voice, 30, 33

W

withdrawal, 21, 26, 35
workflow, 24, 45
workspace, 21, 24, 34, 39
workstation, 10, 30, 33